A DOCTOR IN PRACTICE

A DOCTOR IN PRACTICE

Geoffrey Hale and Nesta Roberts

Routledge & Kegan Paul
London and Boston

First published in 1974
by Routledge & Kegan Paul Ltd
Broadway House, 68–74 Carter Lane,
London EC4V 5EL and
9 Park Street,
Boston, Mass. 02108, USA

Photoset and printed
in Great Britain by
REDWOOD BURN LIMITED
Trowbridge & Esher

ISBN 0 7100 7745 9

Library of Congress Catalog Card No. 73–86573

To the future of the National Health Service, to the general practitioners of this country in whose hands it largely rests, and to the memory of its founder, Aneurin Bevan, Minister of Health, 1945 to 1951

CONTENTS

PREFACE

What is it like to be a doctor? More specifically, what was it like to be a doctor in Britain during an epoch extending over forty years, from leeches to lasers, which saw medicine revolutionised by the discovery of antibiotics and society transformed by the birth of the Welfare State?

This book, which is neither polemic nor apologia, tries to answer those questions by examining and recording as faithfully as possible the experiences and reactions of one practitioner whose active career coincides with that eventful period. Since he is a real, not an imaginary, figure, the approach is necessarily biographical, but the biography is less that of a man than that of a vocation. The vocation is the one in which the art of medicine can reach its peak – general practice.

In the narrative all individuals who held or hold known positions of any kind have been given their real names. So have all connected with St Thomas's Hospital, except that the convention of referring to Sisters by the names of their wards has been observed.

Pseudonyms have been used for all but two of the other characters. They are Dr Scott, of Windsor, who may be said to have started the whole thing, and Mrs Chitty, who demonstrated so vividly to her small pupils how the earth turned on its axis. There is no logical reason for this exception. It was just that neither of these two would come alive under any name other than their own.

The authors wish to thank the Editors of *Lancet* and the *British Medical Journal* for permission to quote from correspondence and articles published in their respective journals, and the Secretary of the Medical School of the University of Oxford for permission to quote from an article on Sir William Osler, written by F. G. Hobson for the *Medical School Gazette*.

CHAPTER 1

HOME AND BACKGROUND: 'I'M GOING TO BE A DOCTOR'

Sixty-two years on, the Doctor is perfectly clear about the moment when he decided on what was to be his life's work. He was three years old; he was ill with bronchitis; Dr Scott had come all the way from Windsor to Slough to visit him, and he had come in a motor car. The motor car may have clinched the matter. They were not common in the Thames Valley in 1908. But Dr Scott was nice too, kind and cheerful and healthy looking. The little boy liked him very much, and – perhaps this was the first manifestation of what was to be a notably unvindictive nature – continued to like him even after Dr Scott had ordered a Sanitas bath to cleanse him after measles. A doctor was certainly a good thing to look forward to being, but, for the present, he was rather fully occupied with being a patient. He was continually catching colds which ended in bronchitis, so that his earliest medical memories were of his mother preparing linseed poultices by candle-light, of cottonwool chest protectors, and a steam kettle on the hob, and inhalations of friar's balsam. Decades later the Doctor was to pass on his mother's method to such of his patients as still practised inhalation, teaching them that to wrap a stiff towel round the steaming jug, like a funnel, then put one's mouth over it and breathe in gently, was quite as effective and a lot more comfortable than being totally extinguished beneath the towel. He himself was extinguished only during the perilous operation of Airing the Room, when he was sheeted like the dead until the windows were safely closed again.

Possibly both techniques had been instituted by his father, who had put up his plate at Eton in 1894, in the most auspicious conditions for building up a good family practice. He had been born, brought up and educated at Eton; his own father, at this time, was still an Eton housemaster; his father-

1

in-law had been another before going on to become, successively, Headmaster of Cheltenham, Professor of Greek at Durham University and a canon of the cathedral.

'He was a responsible, well-mannered man, generous to his poor patients', recalls the son who never knew him. To an age mildly besotted by the marvels of chemotherapy it may not sound an impressive recommendation for a member of a scientific profession. But at a period when the only substances that could be administered to a patient which acted, and which could be seen to act, were laxatives – hence the early insistence on purging – so that all a physician could do was to build up the general constitution, alleviate symptoms and inspire the patient with the determination to get well, the qualities that his father possessed were important ones. They enhanced the popularity and regard that he enjoyed in a community where he was already well known. He did his rounds on a bicycle, hiring a fly in particularly bad weather, worked fifty hours a week, or less, in summer, and perhaps sixty-five a week in winter, and, by 1904, had increased his annual earnings from the £600 or so of his first year in practice to £2,000, a considerable sum for the time.

In December of that year came a dramatic illustration of what was implied by the lack of specific remedies in the armoury of the physician of the period. He caught scarlet fever from one of his patients, and septicaemia developed. He died aged thirty-nine, leaving a widow, a son aged nine and a daughter aged six. A shocked and grieving local community subscribed £700 towards a memorial fund, the income from which was to be used to provide convalescent holidays for the needy, and which, to this day, provides occasional comforts for patients recommended by the district nurse. Six months after his father's death, the Doctor, his second son and namesake, was born.

By that time the family had left the house in Eton High Street for a modest semi-detached on a private housing estate at Slough. The household was augmented by an unmarried aunt who had come to give moral and material support to her sister-in-law, and possibly, also, to act as chaperone at a time when conventional society was apt to raise at least one eyebrow at women who lived alone, unless they adopted a way of life suitable for an enclosed nun. In 1905, for the middle

2

classes, modesty was a relative concept. The rent of the 'semi' was £50 a year, but, like all the thirty or so houses on the estate, which had been built about sixty years previously, it had the appurtenances of gentility. There was a half-basement planned for servants, with a row of clapper bells connecting with the principal rooms, and, until the outbreak of the First World War, there were, in fact, two living-in servants, though nanny and nursemaid had had to go. The basement, like the landing and corridors, was lit by fishtail gas burners. Most bedrooms had oil lamps and candles. Only the hall and the first floor bedrooms enjoyed the modified brilliance of incandescent globes. The coach house, with stabling for two, remained untenanted, as did those of all the neighbours, until the Army billeted its horses there during the First World War. But there were private approach roads guarded by lodges which housed the estate workers, and several acres of communal garden sloping down to the kingcups and moorhens of the water meadows where the M4 now runs. One could glimpse the towers of Eton; and the Royal Standard, printed against the sky, gave regular assurance that the King was in his castle and, by extension, God in his heaven.

Privilege was the more inalienable for being unconscious; reputation survived the grave. The child became used to hearing family friends speak well of his father, and himself began to be proud of having had a parent whom people looked up to – proud not because his father had been an important person, but because, clearly, he had been a good, kind man. Long afterwards he was to say that, by possessing the image of a father which could be adjusted to meet his needs, he had been spared all the troubles of sons who had difficulty in living up to their fathers. At this time his own often-repeated announcement that he, too, was going to be a doctor was received, if not very seriously, always with pleasure. Living as he did in a household of women – his elder brother, being at boarding school, hardly figured in it – he had not, indeed, much idea of what else people did do except be schoolmasters and parsons.

The beginning of education did nothing to remedy that situation. After pothooks and hangers at home, there was a short period of morning lessons with the wife of an Eton master, in company with two other small boys, both of whom were to be

Cambridge contemporaries and one of whom was to become his brother-in-law. Here, there were glimpses of the wider shores of learning. Who could fail to thrill, like Galileo, to the notion of the earth's turning on its axis when Mrs Chitty drove a pencil through an orange at a slight diagonal, rotated it, then royally tossed the orange into the waste-paper basket? But there were still no males over the age of about eight, and the next move, to a governess who lived with her elderly mother on the far side of Windsor, was no help, though it did provide the adventure of an unaccompanied bus journey.

A harsher world broke in for the first time during a wait at a bus stop in an interval of one of those journeys. A gang of urchins – there must have been at least three of them – surrounded the small boy, demanding money. He was terrified. Nothing in the upbringing of a little gentleman had been a preparation for such a situation. Besides, as he explained to the gangsters, he had no money, only twopence for his bus fare home. He offered them instead an invitation to a children's party which he chanced to have in his pocket. It was already out of date, but it had a picture on the front and the gangsters seemed satisfied. He fled. The episode indicated that it was more than time for the toughening course of the Wick.

The Wick was near Brighton. The climate was bracing in every sense, and sixty little gentlemen were prepared mainly for Winchester; the emphasis accordingly was on discipline, good manners and the classics. Mr Thring, the headmaster, was severe, with one eye and a walrus moustache. His sister and adjutant was strict and given to trumpeting: 'X! X! Hold yourself properly!' at a small boy who, since his bronchitis now usually ended in asthma, tended to hunch his shoulders. Looking back, in charity, the Doctor does not think that she was really unkind, merely devoted to the Manners Makyth Man notion, even if, objectively, the results were much the same. He came to feel, also, that there could be worse preliminaries to life as a GP than that early insistence on courtesy.

The rigours of the first term were softened by the help of a kind, fatherly little boy who appeared in the school lists as Butler II, but even the former Minister of Education and Chancellor of the Exchequer and present Master of Trinity could not temper the miseries of broken chilblains which afflicted most of the little gentlemen at The Wick each winter.

There was some central heating in some parts of the building, but the underlying principle was that low temperatures were conducive to robust moral fibre and that cold water was sovereign in almost all circumstances. Every morning, immediately after the seven o'clock rising bell, Mr Thring donned a mackintosh and made a round of the dormitories, collecting his charges in batches of twenty, who, towels over their arms and dressing-gowns to cover their shivering nakedness, followed him to a bathroom whose window, summer and winter alike, stood wide open. There Mr Thring, warmly waterproofed, established himself on a dais while, one by one, the boys shed their dressing-gowns, stepped up in front of him, raised their arms above their heads and pirouetted three times while he directed the cold shower on to them. Then, dripping, they retreated to the edge of the dais and took three deep breaths before they were allowed to dry themselves, put on their dressing-gowns and return to their dormitories. If, despite all that conditioning, anybody fell ill, the doctor came and always prescribed the same fizzy medicine that looked like champagne. It was to be years before our Doctor learned just how unlike champagne it tasted. He had it for mumps, chicken pox and whooping cough. For what, with hindsight, he recognised as a sub-acute attack of appendicitis, the doctor was, of course, not called, since at that time it was recognised that little boys were liable to stomach-ache and there was no occasion to fuss over it. The whooping cough epidemic provided a variation, in that some of the boys – whether the inspiration came from the doctor or from Miss Thring – wore chopped-up garlic inside their socks, the idea being that the oils would be absorbed through the soles of the feet and excreted through the breath, doing something fortifying to the lungs en route. There was sensible evidence that they were excreted. But perhaps the régime did, after all, promote the fitness at which it aimed, because, when Spanish influenza hit The Wick in the summer of 1918, the boys went down like a pack of cards, but nobody was very ill. For the Doctor the immunity so gained proved valuable when he went on to Shrewsbury in September. By then the epidemic had travelled west and, in his first term, he sang in the choir at the funerals of three schoolfellows, an experience which largely passed over his head.

5

There were cold showers at Shrewsbury, too, though the procedure was less picturesque. You left your dormitory, mother-naked, to proceed along a corridor to the bathroom. There you waited your turn to stand on a small platform which sank under your weight to release an icy douche. Still, the Doctor never had chilblains. It was something to be placed on the credit side of six years during which, while climbing from the bottom of the school to the sixth form, he remembers having been, for much of the time, idle and bored – idle chiefly because bored.

Thanks to the high educational standards set by Mr Thring, he did not cover any new ground for his first two years at Shrewsbury, and even after that he found only two masters whose teaching was stimulating. Strictly, perhaps, only one, since the maths master was stimulating mostly because he lost his temper. The Doctor was no good at football or cricket; running, which was something of a fetish, he mercifully escaped because of his asthma. What, from the beginning, he looked forward to was rowing. It was the natural choice for a boy whose father had been in the Eton Eight and got a Cambridge trial cap, whose maternal grandfather had stroked the Cambridge boat and whose great-great-uncle had rowed in the first Boat Race. He was just about old enough to join the Boat Club when a day came on which he was one of three boys to report to Matron with an upset stomach.

They were seen by the school doctor, who prescribed castor oil all round. His was the appendix, and it burst that afternoon, though nobody knew it. He was kept in bed and seen regularly by the doctor, but there was no diagnosis, and it was a fortnight before a surgeon was called, to pronounce that he had peritonitis and was in urgent need of an operation. 'It wasn't necessarily his fault', says the Doctor now, showing impeccable professional solidarity with the school medico. 'Appendicitis in small boys is notoriously difficult to diagnose.'

The ambulance which took him to the nursing home was horse drawn. He regrets still that he was in no state to notice whether or not it had straw on the floor. There was one operation, there was another operation, there were prayers in the school chapel and there was Napoleon brandy. The brandy had been a legacy to his housemaster. A somewhat emotional bachelor, he had decided it was too precious to drink. It must be kept for saving young lives, and the Doctor's was the first young life to be saved. The brandy was administered, in tea, by the night nurse at 4 a.m. Life-saving or not, it was a comforting interval during a long and sometimes sleepless night. When, at last, his name was taken off the danger list and the prayers in chapel stopped, the Napoleon brandy stopped too, being replaced by Hennessy's Three Star. You could tell the difference even in tea. The liqueur brandy had been a bonus. The incidental trials included the 'anaesthetic eyes' which were a frequent sequel to surgery in the early 1920s, when anaesthesia was still at a relatively primitive stage. The anaesthetist dripped a mixture of ether and chloroform on to a mask until the patient went off, then usually changed to pure ether, and, seated at the head of the operating table, touched the cornea from time to time to see if there was a reflex. Whether because of an accidental splash of ether into the eyes or because the cornea was prodded too enthusiastically, the result was often acute conjunctivitis. You got zinc sulphate drops by way of treatment, otherwise you just waited for it to get better.

All told, the business caused him to miss two terms, made him a passenger for a third and put paid to any idea of rowing for the rest of his school career. But things did begin to improve slightly. School was still dull, and, looking back, he wonders that, from mere tedium, he never got into worse trouble than having to write out a whole book of *Paradise Lost* for having organised a sweep on the Grand National. He took to shooting as an alternative to cricket, chiefly because lying on your stomach on the grass was quite an agreeable way of spending a summer afternoon, and got into the school team that went to Bisley. There was no more Napoleon brandy, but every Sunday evening his housemaster invited half a dozen boys to dinner. It was a social exercise, whose object was to ensure that they would know how to conduct themselves at tables more elaborately appointed than those in the school dining hall, and conversation was painful, but you got a jolly good dinner, and went to bed pleasantly tipsy after the sequence of sherry, claret and port. He got more than his share of invitations because his housemaster suspected that, being fatherless, he would have less opportunity than most of learning what went into which glass, as was indeed true. Not until his older brother came out of the Army to go up to Oxford did alcohol appear on the table at home, and then it was limited to beer.

The serious difference was that, by now, he had given more or less adult consideration to the idea of being a doctor, which he had held unquestioningly since the age of three. What else could one possibly be? Spending one's life in an office was a horrible idea. Schoolmaster? He didn't think he was clever enough, even if the idea had been attractive. A parson was more to his taste, only he did not feel particularly religious or churchy. There were no objections whatsoever to the notion of being a doctor, and all things to be said for it. The concept of 'status' was not one of them, nor was money. Status was what you had, and nothing could take it from you. Obviously, if you were a good doctor you would have more status than if you were a bad one, but there was no question of improving it by becoming one. As for money, so far as he thought about it at all, the doctors he knew seemed to be, if not rich, comfortably off. So he went over to the science side, registered as a medical student and started working for his First MB, which, in those days, could be taken at school. Specialisation was fairly strict. The humanities occupied the least possible place in the time-table and school did not offer much in the way of art and music outside the classroom. Looking back dispassionately over half a century, the Doctor sees himself at this period as a pretty average young blimp, aware of but not involved in the events of the outside world, uninterested in politics and quite incapable of relating social conditions to political policies. When, or if, he thought of things like unemployment, or hunger, or homelessness, he was sorry, as he would have been sorry about any other Act of God which caused suffering, but he accepted that nothing could be done about them, though he would have been ready to give half, or even the whole, of his dinner to a starving individual if one had presented himself. The idea of demonstrating about social conditions, in White-hall or elsewhere, would no more have occurred to him than that of flying to the moon.

People, on the other hand, were beginning to be an object of interest and concern. It was chiefly the insight they gave you into the thoughts and motives and feelings of people that turned him to books in the holidays. All of Hardy, among a good deal else. And there was the business of Emily. Emily was the cook-general at home, the war having cut the effectives of the genteel half-basement by 50 per cent. She had had one illegitimate child when she was engaged by the Doctor's mother, who was considered to be, in about equal proportions, noble and almost dangerously broadminded as a result. Even her charity was strained when Emily went on to have another child. Surprisingly, the man married her, which meant a third child, and deplorable housing in an old Army hut for the family of five. During one holiday the Doctor spent a good deal of time accompanying Emily's husband on the round of agents and local authority officers and small speculative builders. He is even less clear now than he was then about what he could possibly have done to help at the age of seventeen or so, but perhaps an expensive accent was a help in getting a hearing, and, for Emily's husband, even a young gentleman was better than nobody.

In 1924 the academic rat race had not been dreamed of. For Cambridge you had to negotiate Little Go, but that was chiefly a matter of making sure you got up the right book of Ovid. King's, his father's college, required something more, since all its undergraduates were expected to read for honours degrees, but he had managed to get his First MB, and that did the trick. He turned his back on what had been, for him, the Dark Ages – he knew that these were supposed to have been the best years of his life, but he did hope not, even though he would never have thought of questioning the public school ethos – and stepped into the sunlight of his personal Renaissance.

Cambridge was marvellous; there was so much to do and to look at and to be interested in. King's was its heart, its charmed centre. It received a young man who was a self-confessed hearty – only you would have had to be a clot as well as a hearty not to react at all to the beauty of the surroundings and the music in chapel – and sent him out at the end of three years with some elementary notions about the meaning of civilisation, as well as an abiding love of the place. He made friends almost at once, and now, at last, he was able to take up the only sport in which he was interested, rowing. He devoted every spare moment to the river, and was pleased, flattered and satisfied to row in both the Lent and the May boat in his first year. The friends were all 'people like us'. The Etonian monopoly of King's had ended in the 1880s, but public school-boys still made up the large majority of the college. There were people from grammar schools who were up on scholar-ships, but one hardly knew them. They lived mostly in Chetwynd Court, or in an annexe approached by a tunnel under the lane, almost a ghetto really, and sometimes their clothes were a bit different. He was blimpish enough to avoid their company – or was it that he was slightly afraid of it because he did not know how to get on with them? The 'God wod', a group made up largely of Choral Scholars, he tended to laugh at, though nobody could laugh at the Dean, who was their prophet. Milner-White's gifts were so various as to sug-gest that he was several persons in one substance. Besides being priest and historian, he was a disciple of Keynes, and his acumen in economic and financial matters had, it was credibly reported, enabled him to amass a fortune on the Stock Exchange, and give it away. His interests ranged from stained glass to rose growing. All that and a DSO too. The aesthetes, whose trousers were pinker (it was the era of Oxford bags in pastel shades), whose hair was longer than the average, and who had Victorian wax funeral wreaths under glass globes in their rooms, no doubt laughed at the Doctor and his friends.

Medical students, particularly in colleges where they are numerous, tend to be a class apart who are not much sub-jected to the humanising influence which is supposed to be one of the raisons d'être of a university. At King's they were so few that they were absorbed into the normal life of the college.

At that time, 1924-7, medieval austerity and patrician amplitude co-existed. The only form of heating in the Doctor's rooms was a coal fire. His sponge froze regularly on winter nights and there was a legend that a friend, having put a small dental plate in a glass by his bedside, was startled as he was dropping off to sleep by the crack of the glass as the water turned to ice. No water was laid on in undergraduates' rooms. The bedmakers kept washstand jugs filled from a single tap somewhere on the stairs, or in the basement, and baths and lavatories were across one if not two courts, depending upon where one lived. But a gentleman of means could live in the style to which he was accustomed, having dinner, as elaborate

10

as he cared to order, served in his rooms, with College plate to supplement his own silver, and employing a gyp as valet as well as butler. Not being gentlemen of means of that kind, the Doctor and most of his friends availed themselves of the dinner service only on special occasions, like Mays, and looked after their own clothes – in so far as they were looked after.

By today's standards, clothes were formal, nothing more unstudied than flannels and a sports jacket, and always a collar and tie. Shirts as well as suits were bespoke; nevertheless it was said at the time that a gentleman could dress on £20 a year, of which £12 should be spent on his annual suit. The Doctor never spent as much, except during the year when he had his tails made, for the sum of £18. He had £300 a year to cover everything, including vacations, though then, of course, you lived free at home. A three-course dinner in Hall cost three shillings. Lunch, at one-and-six, was a relaxed, agreeable occasion, where an undergraduate might find himself sitting next to a Fellow, or even the Provost, but one could not afford that every day. More often one had bread and cheese in one's rooms. For the same reason, most people got their own breakfasts in their rooms, except when they were in training for the Lents or Mays, when, for a fortnight before the event, they went into Hall for vast rowing breakfasts which started with porridge and went on through fish, and eggs and bacon, to toast and marmalade with quantities of coffee. With those minor economies, the £300 covered everything quite comfortably, 'everything' ranging from a motor-bike and sidecar to chocolate cakes and sponge cakes from FitzBilly's for the fire-lit teas that came after winter afternoons on the river. They were nearly the best part of the day. The absolute best were the coffee parties in people's rooms after Hall. Dons came to them. People like Shepherd and Adcock were not remote figures; they lived in college and you met them on equal terms. Night after night the Doctor sat drinking in talk such as he had never heard in his life. He cannot remember ever contributing to it. It was enough just to be there, and in that brilliant company a little of the gold dust perhaps rubbed off on you.

Gilded or not, he was still quite unconscious politically. The General Strike was a tremendous lark. It was bad luck that, because of labs, he could not go off with his friends to drive engines or unload ships at Hull or London docks. All he did was an occasional patrol on the motor-bike. You trundled up the London road, then returned to report that it was clear and you had seen no strikers. There were a few undergraduates who went off and worked for the TUC. Actually it wasn't all that surprising, because they had been known to be a bit Left and different. It was rather the sort of thing you would expect from chaps at Downing. Nobody held it against them when they came back. The mild scandal in which the Doctor himself was involved, and as a result of which he was sent out of college during his last year – a major social inconvenience as well as being about as close as you could get to being sent down – was mere rowdyism. With fellow members of a college society which held bibulous monthly meetings, he had taken part in a midnight bottle-throwing contest on the back lawn, and some of the bottles went through a couple of windows in Clare, next door. There was no political motive; there was no publicity; the damage was confined to university premises. In short, a far different affair from the 'Garden House' business; but, forty years on or thereabouts, the Doctor was concerned to bring to a better frame of mind a fellow Old Kingsman who thought that undergraduates convicted for their actions during the demonstration should be punished additionally by being sent down. 'Surely you wouldn't turn out your daughter if she brought home an illegitimate baby?'

By this time he was wholly and utterly committed to medicine. Sometimes he was discouraged at the terribly long road he would have to travel to qualification, and wondered if he would ever make it, but he could not even contemplate any other career.

A year before he went down he had to decide to which London hospital he would go on, being left to make up his mind with no suggestions from any of his tutors. The obvious choice was St. George's, where his father and uncle had trained, but, justifiably or not, he had got the idea that it was not what it had been. He liked the kind of people who had already opted for St Thomas's, but the determining factor in his choice was even more personal. Through a friend who was a Choral Scholar he had come to know the widow of a Cambridge doctor, himself a Thomas's man, who had been a contemporary of Dr, later Sir, Maurice Cassidy. The doctor had been looked after there during his terminal illness, and his wife had been greatly impressed both by St Thomas's and by Maurice Cassidy. It sounded a nice place. So, to St Thomas's he applied, in the happy certainty that he would be accepted. So happy that it never even occurred to him that there might be stiff competition or a testing interview. He was asked to see the Medical Secretary, Colonel Thompson, as a follow-up to his application, but he regarded this as ordinary routine, not as something which might decide his acceptance or rejection. They were obviously going to take him, so there was nothing to worry about. They took him.

It was a pity about the work, particularly as he had the Second MB as well as the Natural Sciences Tripos to get through. For one thing, he did not adjust well to having to organise his own work; for another, between the river and those magic evenings of talk, there simply was not the time to fit in all the reading he should have done, though he did not cut lectures, and he attended enough labs to get the necessary signatures. Since King's was not a medical place, he went to other colleges for most of his supervision and tuition, though, for a time, he was lucky enough to go to Sir Joseph Barcroft for physiology. Barcroft, who, while doing research into poison gases during the war, went into a gas chamber to support his conviction that a certain compound was not lethal, was delightful as well as brilliant, so the Doctor was the more regretful that he was not himself clever enough to benefit more fully from what was offered. Human physiology, all the same, was about his favourite subject; it was not simply interesting, it was fun. But, probably because his interest in medicine was essentially that of an embryonic physician, he could not beat up much enthusiasm for the detailed anatomy which was required for the Second MB – far too detailed, he still thinks, for those who do not intend to specialise in surgery.

He left Cambridge in 1927, after three idle, well-spent years, having got a Third, and lucky at that, in the Tripos and clocked up two failures in the Second MB, coming down in anatomy each time.

CHAPTER 2

MEDICAL SCHOOL:
TEACHERS AND TAUGHT

As it happened, that twice-failed Second MB was to pay dividends. The first accrued from a viva at which the examiner's attitude suggested that he might have been trying to inch up a candidate who had put in a border-line paper.

'What do you think that is?' he asked, handing over a jar containing an anatomical specimen which was intended to be the starting point for an extended discussion. The Doctor was on his fourth or fifth increasingly wild guess when a gentle voice said: 'Suppose you look at the label.' And there it was, clear to see. It was humiliating, but it taught you. The way to qualification was studded with examinations, and discussing specimens in jars often figured in them. The more abstruse ones were often labelled, for the benefit of the examiners, who might have been excused for forgetting parts of the curriculum which were twenty or thirty years behind them, and the Doctor, by then a more experienced candidate, always began by turning them up for verification. It might have earned him an extra mark or two for resource: certainly it seldom failed to draw a sympathetic smile from examiners.

For the moment it was no use pretending that the prospect of sitting the wretched examination for the third time was anything other than a cloud on the further horizon, but it was not allowed to shadow the summer vacation. The Doctor's older brother and a friend who was a psychologist intended to sail down the east coast and west to the Isles of Scilly; he and a Cambridge friend were invited to join them.

In the 1920s amateur sailors did not have the monopoly of coastal waters. There were still working craft under sail in the Channel, notably the marvellous Thames barges, which went down to Portland to load stone, and which could sail, it seemed, almost into the wind. The party's own seamanship

14

was responsible, according to the standard of the time, which is to say that navigation was competent and the sea and the weather were held in respect, but safety devices were limited to a few flares and a standard cork ring or two to chuck after anybody who went overboard. In this, undoubtedly, they were in the same case as the companies of the coasters which they encountered, but the lack of personal life-jackets still gives a retrospective twinge of guilt to the Doctor, who, in later years, was to be intimately connected with the development of the RNLI life-jacket. Admittedly, those life-jackets which were available at the time were both cumbersome and not particularly efficient.

The round trip lasted an idyllic month. It was the second time that the Doctor had sailed with the psychologist, who was currently working on the new theory of accident-proneness. He was an enthusiast and a great talker. The Doctor remained as good a listener as he had been at Cambridge. Only later was he to realise how much of the fundamental principles of psychology he had absorbed during those two voyages.

There were a few weeks at home before work started. The social historians remember 1927 for dole queues and hunger marches, but life in the Thames Valley had not changed radically. You played tennis, and pursued girls with more or less ardour, and, in the evenings, sometimes went up to Maidenhead on the motor-bike, to dance at Skindle's, or at Murray's, where there was a glass floor lit from underneath. Coming back one night along the old Bath road, whose every bump cast a long shadow in the wavering light of the acetylene lamp, the Doctor was on top of one of them before he realised that it was a body. The sidecar went over one leg. Fortunately the sidecar was empty that night, because the girl of the moment lived at Maidenhead. He pulled up and went back. A man was walking along the side of the road. 'Excuse me,' said the Doctor, 'I think I ran over you.' 'Yes', replied the victim. 'Thank you for waking me up.' The two nations confronted each other in the private universe of the small hours, the tall young medical student, with the gleam of his patent leather shoes a little dimmed by the dust of the Bath road, and the unemployed man from the West Country who had dropped flat out in his tracks. The man had had a letter with bad news from his sister, he said, and he was walking up to London 'to save her honour'. Looking back, the Doctor cannot remember having been particularly struck by such an illustration of the general injustice of life. He never was a great one for analysing his emotions and reactions. Instead, he said: 'Get in!' and drove the man up to London. It did not seem polite to ask direct questions about his sister, so he never did find out what had put her honour in jeopardy, nor how his passenger proposed to save it.

He went up to St Thomas's early, to get settled before term began. There was no problem about accommodation. An aunt, his father's sister, had married, as his second wife, Sir Thomas Chitty, Senior Master of the Court of Chancery. Sir Thomas's family having grown up and left home, the large house in Kensington opened its doors to a stream of nephews and nieces, and the Doctor, in his turn, was invited to live there while he was at St Thomas's. It was a far cry from student digs to the amenities of No 48, Queen's Gate Gardens, with its five indoor servants, plus a man who came in for boots and odd jobs. Later, the Doctor was to regret a little that living there had prevented him from taking much part in the social life of the hospital. At the time there was no question about it. Economically he was not in a position to turn down a free billet, even it it would not have been ungracious to do so.

Since he had no living expenses and went home for weekends, his allowance came down from the £300 of Cambridge to between £150 and £200 a year, from which he had to pay £50 hospital dues and buy the necessary books. There was enough left over to run the three-wheeled Morgan which he had inherited from his brother, and which he garaged on hospital property for 2s. 6d. a week. At that time unused warehouses behind the students' club provided all the parking space needed by the minority of students who possessed some kind of vehicle, in contrast to the present day, when most are mechanised and the hospital can provide almost no parking space. Socially speaking the car was a great improvement on the bike. It was a bit much to ask a girl to come to a dance in a sidecar. You did ask her, of course, and, usually, she came, but it was more seemly to put a hood over her. After that there was not much to spare, and the Doctor never did find the £20 to pay for the microscope which students were recommended to buy. It was an awful lot of money to part with at one go, particularly when he did not want to be a pathologist, so he went on taking turns at the hospital microscopes.

In those days, St Thomas's was still housed in the building which Queen Victoria had opened in 1871. It was so large that, for some years, it was only partly occupied, and, in 1879, paying patients had been admitted in an effort to meet the cost of 'over building'. The most recent addition was the students' club on the opposite side of Lambeth Road, which replaced a dreary collection of Army huts that had previously served that purpose. The new club was on the grandiose scale, well furnished and offering full West End amenities, including thirty or forty bed-sitting rooms, some of which were reserved for casualty officers and house surgeons and physicians of special departments who did not have to live in the hospital itself. There were stewards in striped jackets to staff the excellent ground floor dining-room, and the exemplary Hutton, in tail coat with shiny crested buttons, in the porter's lodge. Had the club, like the hospital of 1871, been overbuilt? Within a year the West End atmosphere had gone. The dining-room had been handed over to a firm of caterers, and Nippy-type waitresses replaced the stewards. Hutton remained, a survivor from a nobler age.

There were about 350 students, of whom forty or fifty each year came up from the universities (which, effectively, meant Oxbridge), the same number from the hospital Medical School, which they had entered direct from school – almost exclusively public schools, whether major or minor – and a few from overseas. The Medical School entry were part of London University and took its degrees; the rest, if they aimed for higher degrees, took those of their own university. Since entry via the Medical School shortened the training time by a year, money usually dictated the choice at a period when there were no student grants to supplement such scholarships as were available. Almost all lived on allowances from their parents; probably for that reason, in contrast to today, virtually no students were married. The men from overseas were mostly Africans. The Doctor remembers no trace of racial feeling among the students, but remembers, too, that it no more occurred to him to make friendly overtures to them, over and above the normal day to day civilities, than it had occurred to

17

him to make similar approaches to the Northern Grammar School boys at King's. He had plenty of friends; it would have seemed unnatural to go out of his way to take up with people with whom he had nothing in common.

About the same proportion of students as that of today, 15 to 20 per cent, were doctors' children, which is to say doctors' sons. Doctors' daughters did not appear until after 1948, when the NHS required the teaching hospitals to take a quota of women students. As is also true today, they tended to have a slightly higher proportion of failures and drop-outs than students from non-medical families, which proves nothing either way about heredity. It was, and remains, related to the fact that the sons of doctors, particularly of GPs, tend to be pressurised into following their fathers into a profession for which they may have no real taste or aptitude. Lucky are those who find out their mistake early.

All but the outstandingly brilliant and confident took the 'conjoint', or MRCS (Membership of the Royal College of Surgeons) and LRCP (Licentiate of the Royal College of Physicians) diplomas, which authorised them to practise, as well as the university degrees in medicine and surgery, MB and B.Chir, or BS at London University. The former had the advantage of being held every quarter, unlike the university examinations, which took place only twice a year, so that one failure did not keep you back so long. Thomas's disapproved stongly of students' taking the LMSSA, the diploma of the Society of Apothecaries, which, being reputedly the least exacting examination of all, was regarded as a back door into the profession. Nevertheless, it was occasionally resorted to as the help of the perishing, usually those whose means, or whose families' means ran out before they had got the more usual qualifications. The world being less demanding than the hospital, some built up successful medical careers on the foundations of the LMSSA alone.

Living with the family meant that the Doctor worked a good deal harder than he might otherwise have done. Without actually being beastly about it, his aunt and uncle were firmly encouraging that he should get down to his books once dinner was over. Besides, while there was no rule about the number of times one could sit the Second MB, it was too expensive to keep on failing. He passed it quite comfortably in December and, in January, entered the hospital to start medicine proper.

Life was transformed. He had always found it easier to learn from people, from talking and listening and doing, than from books, and now he was working three-dimensionally nearly all the time. Now, too, he reaped another advantage from those early failures. Because he was three months behind his university contemporaries, he came into the hospital to do his terms in its various departments in a group of only four, instead of the normal dozen or so. It meant that one had three times as many patients to study, and, inevitably, that one came in for more individual attention from teachers. The other three had not got left behind through being idle. They were clever young men who had stayed on at the Medical School to take the Primary FRCS, on the way to higher degrees in surgery. All later became consultants.

In the light of experience the first three months of preliminary medicine would probably have seemed rather dull, but, coming to it new, the Doctor found it absorbing. The students were taught to percuss chests, and listen to hearts, and test reflexes, the whole routine of a proper and careful examination, including the taking of notes and the writing out of a full history, personal and medical, several pages long. Learning the routine of examination and becoming a competent examiner are, needless to say, not the same thing. Only experience can teach a doctor when 'abnormalities' are simply variations on the norm. It was all done in one medical ward, where the patients did not seem unduly disturbed by the process, under three excellent teachers, John Forest Smith, Harold Gardiner Hill and Isaac Jones. There was another equally stimulating teacher, B.W. Williams, for the surgical half of the introductory course, which was spent in the Casualty department.

In the 1930s, when only wage-earners were eligible for medical benefits, Casualty implied something more comprehensive than the accidents and emergencies of today, though these had their due place. One of the Doctor's memories is of seeing, on a morning of freezing fog, eight Metropolitan policemen sitting in a row in the department, each holding an arm which had suffered a Colles fracture in a fall on the ice-bound roads. St Thomas's was the collective GP for the mothers of Lambeth and their children, a responsibility which it assumed willingly. In return, the people of Lambeth had affection as well as respect for the hospital, even though it might be mingled with trepidation. 'Stoppit!' a mother was heard to say to a bawling three-year-old whom she was lugging along Lambeth Palace Road. 'Stoppit, I say! If you don't stoppit I'll take you to the hospital, and once you get there you'll have a job to get out.'

Everything came into the long, tiled hall, with its rows of wooden benches, where, as in a swimming pool, women were directed to the right and men to the left: measles and mumps and chicken pox; stomach-aches that might be appendicitis, and ear-aches that might be mastoids; and bad sore throats, every one of which had to be regarded as a potential diphtheria until a swab had proved it innocent. In an era when there were no preventive jabs and the only treatment was anti-toxin pumped in during the early stages of the disease, diphtheria was a killer, responsible for 1,800 deaths in the average year. A membrane in the throat could obstruct breathing: when that happened a quick tracheotomy – making a slit in the windpipe and inserting a breathing tube – had to be done in Casualty, though the Doctor knew of only one during his time, and did not see that. Diphtheria and scarlet fever were sent to the fever hospital quick: of the non-infectious cases requiring more prolonged or elaborate treatment than could be given on the spot some were admitted, others sent to the local authority hospital in Brook Street, now Brook Drive, Lambeth. The gulf between voluntary and local authority hospitals, as expressed in staff and amenities, was wide indeed in the pre-NHS period. The patients were quite well aware of it, and disliked being relegated to what they considered a sub-standard establishment.

The students learned to open abscesses, and give injections, and administer gas – the only anaesthetic used for the minor procedures which were carried out in Casualty – and even pull out teeth. The department was staffed by eight newly qualified young doctors, supervised by a senior, and since every patient was seen by one or other of them, the students had no real responsibility. This, in passing, is the first appearance of a word which is to crop up often in the Doctor's recollections, used always in the context of something to be desired and sought for, rather than something alarming or oppressive to be as far as possible avoided. But the students were actively and usefully employed during a day which lasted from 9 a.m. until 6.30 p.m.

Much of their time was spent hot-fomenting and bandaging under the tutelage of Sister Casualty, a splendid, bustling, motherly Amazon who did not spare students, found time amid all the to-ing and fro-ing to sort out the cares and troubles of the patients as well as to deal with their physical ills, and favoured practical remedies for all problems. It was reported that her successor once consulted the log book for advice on dealing with difficulties, and, under 'Brought in Dead', found: 'If relatives appear worried or distressed, give them a cup of hot tea.' Perhaps it was as valid a counsel as any for a situation which essentially has to be played by ear. Like most of his fellow students, the Doctor began by being a little afraid of Sister Casualty, went on to laugh at her privately, and later, as a casualty officer, became devoted to her.

At a period when antibiotics were unknown and when the sparse diet that went with widespread unemployment meant that natural resistance was apt to be low, the department seethed with local infection. Cuts and thorn pricks went bad; the trouble often spread to the bone, bits of which came out through the wound, and it was fairly common to have to re-move the top joint of a finger. Boils and carbuncles and whit-lows and abscesses and impetigo arrived in their battalions. Students were warned against touching their faces while doing dressings, because of transferring infection, but you had to be more than human not to do so in the room where half a dozen of them worked, because the cotton wool dust stuck to your nose and tickled intolerably. After eight weeks the Doctor got impetigo. It sent him home for another six, during which two hours of every day were taken up by treatment in-volving first sousing the affected area in Eusol, which stank, then plastering it with yellow, messy ointment, known in the hospital as ung. hyd. nit. dil. which today is virtually unheard of. Shaving was out; he had to trim his beard with scissors.

Thank goodness, when he got back to the hospital, he had done with Casualty for the time being! Now each student was attached to the 'firm' of one of the honorary physicians or sur-geons. A firm consisted of the Chief, an Assistant Physician or

21

surgeon, who was also a senior consultant, and the group of students for whom they were responsible. Was it due to the good offices of that mutual friend at Cambridge or was it sheer luck that the Doctor found himself assigned to the firm of Dr Maurice Cassidy, which looked after Arthur, a male medical ward, and half Victoria, a women's medical ward? There were fifteen beds, with tall windows between them, on either side of the rectangular rooms, each opening on to a balcony looking over the river. There were no partitions or curtains, only screens for privacy. In the eighteenth century every bed had had its semi-circle of curtains in winter. No doubt they were swept away by Florence Nightingale as being liable to harbour germs. Today there are curtains once more.

Sister made the first impact. Sister Casualty had been a dynamic schoolmistress. Sister Arthur was tall, blonde, dignified and beautiful, a wonderful nurse who was adored by her patients and who seemed incapable of being discomposed. She had come to St Thomas's from VAD service in the First World War, and, after leaving it, became matron of big military hospitals during the Second World War. No one who met her during a distinguished career, which culminated in the General Secretaryship of the International Council of Nurses, could have suspected that she had come into the profession by accident – at the outbreak of the 1914 war she had just qualified for Oxford. Now she made clear to the new brood of students that they must not make a clatter in the ward, which meant having rubber heels fitted to their shoes, that they must behave discreetly and that if they disturbed a patient's bed during examination, they must remake it comfortably before leaving. The Doctor vowed allegiance to her on sight, but, at that stage, did not dream that, forty years on, he would still have the honour of counting her as a friend. Sister Arthur, who was good at spotting future winners among the successive generations of students and young doctors who padded through her ward, was fairly soon confident that she had one in this young man, who, from the beginning, did not have to be taught that patients were people, not cases. She could not foresee that, mentally, she was marking favourably her future GP.

'Wasn't he a good exam passer?' she was to ask long afterwards, with a detached interest that seemed to give examinations a legitimate but far from inflated place in the business of becoming a doctor. 'How curious, when, both as a student and as a young doctor, his work was always impeccable.'

Sister Victoria, who was near retiring age, was a far different character, not always at her best with students, though the Doctor got on very well with her. On her ward she walked the delicate line that divides inspiration from eccentricity, and a slight speech impediment, something between a lisp and a whistle, which came and went, added savour to sayings which were to become part of hospital folklore ('Keep your eyes on the shtars, Nursh, and polish the urine glashes to the glory of God!').

The nurses made curiously little impression as individuals: one did not even know their names. For that matter, the hospital custom of referring to Sisters by the names of their wards meant that you seldom knew their names either. In later life it could make for awkward moments before you established that 'my niece Imogen', whom an acquaintance credited you with having known, had been Sister Medical Outpatients. Whatever hospital fiction might lead one to suppose went on in other places, there was strictly no hob-nobbing with Nightingales, who were as closely guarded as the postulants whom in many ways they resembled. To be seen having so much as a pleasant conversation with one meant that a ward sister, or one of the blue bodyguard from Matron's office would be down on the poor girl like a ton of bricks. Taking the matter further just wasn't worth the trouble it would have given you and probably got her into. In this the Doctor was perhaps a little unenterprising, or it may have been that, already, his affections were beginning to be engaged elsewhere. One of his contemporaries succeeded in marrying a Nightingale – true, he had been admitted to City Ward with a carbuncle on his bottom, and relations were cemented over the daily dressings. Another actually married a Sister.

This rather shocked the Doctor. He had never thought of Sisters in that light; it seemed no more than one would have expected that the marriage did not work out very well. Sisters were over thirty – or was it just that, what with one thing and another, they *looked* over thirty by the time they made the grade? During Dame Alicia Lloyd Still's reign as Matron,

Sisters had to wear their hair long, because it was held that the intricately ruched yards of net making up the artefact that is a St Thomas's Sister's cap would not sit gracefully on a bob or shingle, still less an Eton crop, and they might not be Roman Catholics (both rules have long been abolished). The question whether they might be black or coloured did not arise, since, though there were a few Nightingales who came from European countries, the Doctor remembers none who was dark-skinned.

His unawareness of the student nurses as individuals meant that he had no idea of the rigours to which they were subjected during training. Even if he had known, he would have accepted it as part of the existing state of affairs, just as he accepted that nurses, but not medical students or doctors, should have to attend the hospital chapel regularly and take part in the prayers conducted by Sister with which every ward day began and ended. It was like school; the trials you endured when you were a fag or a probationer made you all the more appreciative when you got into the Sixth or became a Sister.

For students, too, the régime recalled school. Each of them had nine or ten patients to examine and look after and write up. The House Physician was a benevolent monitor, who guided your steps and taught you a lot of preliminary medicine. The Registrar – at that time there was only one medical and one surgical Registrar for the whole hospital – who watched over your notes was your housemaster. The Headmaster was the Resident Assistant Physician, with whom the students had little to do. He was the person to whom housemen turned when the Chief was not there.

The day began with a lecture in the Medical School from 9 to 10 a.m. For the next two hours the students were on the wards, then back to the Medical School for another lecture, or practical work, from 12 noon until 1 p.m. Afternoons began in the post mortem room and continued in out-patient clinics, except on the two, or possibly three, days when the 'honoraries' did their ward rounds, which lasted from 2 to 4 p.m. It was little more than ten years after the epoch which had been sharply criticised by Dr F.G. Hobson, Consultant Physician to the United Oxford Hospitals, in a memoir on Sir William Osler, Regius Professor of Medicine at Oxford from 1904-19, who, at the time of his death, was described by the *Lancet* as 'the greatest personality in the medical world'. Dr Hobson, returning to his work at St Thomas's in 1917, after war service, found distasteful the spectacle of 'Physicians, in particular, conducting their teaching rounds in frock coats, pin stripe trousers, and wearing top hats, their diamond tie pins and gold watch chains glinting in the sunlight . . . here were our teachers exhibiting all the crude paraphernalia of social distinction and wealth to humble, poverty stricken and ailing members of their own community.' He went on to contrast the atmosphere during Osler's teaching rounds at the Radcliffe Infirmary with 'The near complete absence of humanity in the handling of patients in this and other major London hospitals.'

In the interval top hats and gold watch chains had gone out. Only two of the 'Honoraries' appeared in morning coats, Dallas Ross, who, since he was an analyst, would anyhow have been considered eccentric by the students, and Walter Howarth, in Ear, Nose and Throat, a short man who might have felt that tails and a topper added a cubit to his stature. Rounds, nevertheless, remained an impressive ceremony. House Physicians and Surgeons, with attendant students, assembled to await the Chief, who arrived in a chauffeur-driven saloon of the type which, today, would be described as vintage. Cassidy's Minerva, though, in fact, the only one of its kind, was typical of 'Honoraries' cars. Sister joined the entourage when the procession reached the ward. At each bed the House Physician or Surgeon normally gave a brief résumé of the case, and the student, known as the clerk, who was responsible for that patient, then read out his full notes, perhaps to be checked if they were over-long, and certain to be asked his opinion of the case. Other students would then be questioned and post-graduates might ask questions. Sometimes the Chief would examine a patient himself. Dr Cassidy always did this on his first visit after the patient's admission.

If the Doctor would have been ready to contest the reproach about the 'near complete absence of humanity in the handing of patients', it was primarily because the hospital made its first imprint on him through Cassidy and wonderful Sister Arthur. Any patient who was looked after by that combination would feel that the stars in their courses were fighting for him. Later the Doctor was to discover that there were consultants and consultants. Some frightened their patients, some humiliated them, some managed virtually to ignore the patient who was the object of the current exercise while at the same time being rude and aggressive in questioning students. The Doctor, who was an observant young man, soon began to notice the difference between physicians and surgeons. The former, almost without exception, were more understanding and helpful and sympathetic. Surgeons were not always able to give the moral support a patient needed after an operation. Really, they were just efficient mechanics, or 'therapeutic technicians', to borrow somebody's phrase. Later, more charitably, he began to think that the war might have been at least partly responsible for their attitude. It had given surgery a tremendous lift, and its practitioners were naturally inclined to be pleased with themselves. Many of the staff had spent their formative years in the Army, dealing with enormous numbers, when they had had to be brusque to get through the work. And the Army of 1914 was still, in spirit, the Army of the nineteenth century, with flogging still in living memory, in which officers treated other ranks much as shooting men treat their gun dogs. They saw that they were adequately fed and lodged, but they would not have thought of giving them an explanation or a reason for any order. Even in civilian life, doctors in general believed that the working classes were not sufficiently intelligent to understand explanations, so there was no point in telling patients why they were being subjected to any procedure. For that matter, they were lucky if they were even told what was going to happen. All the same, the Doctor would have liked to know if those chaps behaved like that with their private patients. Later still, as an established practitioner, with some experience of sitting in on consultants' clinics during refresher courses, he came to accept that there would always be a certain number of immature, inadequate personalities who behaved aggressively to people temporarily in their power, whether patients or students.

In fact St Thomas's, then as now, had a good reputation for treating its patients with courtesy and consideration. The standard was set by the Nightingale School of Nursing. To the specific instruction that they were to treat patients as if they were guests in their own house its young ladies added the qualities deriving from the fact that, for the most part, they were, to use the archaic term, gentlewomen. Their attitude influenced the Doctor from the beginning in his approach to patients. That of Dr Maurice Cassidy made an even greater impression. The reality enhanced the picture which he had built up from hearsay at Cambridge, and which had been largely responsible for his choosing St Thomas's for his medical education. Cassidy was a big, rather shy man who did not find it necessary to exude charm and vitality but who, on the other hand, was never pompous. His dignity came from unfailing good manners, and his rapport with his patients, who sensed in him a genuine desire to get to the bottom of their troubles without being hurried, was founded on his great respect for them.

'He *listened* to them, and I couldn't help seeing how much he learned from what they told him' recalled his pupil towards the end of his own career, during which a patient once described the Doctor as 'the most creative listener in the business'. Dr Maurice Cassidy treated his patients, that is to say, as human beings, and taught his students to do the same. He was an extremely good, careful physician, outstanding on hearts: his students learned to recognise the evidence of early heart disease and when to suspect the deterioration which might lead to a coronary thrombosis. He was already teaching on the electrocardiograph which, for the first time, made possible accurate, measurable assessments of the severity of heart affections. One of its benefits was that no longer would patients suffering merely from nervous palpitation be labelled DAH (Disordered Action of the Heart) and kept in bed for life.

'He was too honest and careful and sincere to be a fashionable doctor', according to our Doctor, who is probably unaware of the distaste for all implied by that term which his tone conveyed, but he had a large private practice which he ran from his large house in Montagu Square. There he entertained his housemen and students at dinner parties where you got the whole works, from caviare to champagne. There were even girls of your own age among the guests, for, on these occasions, the boss imported his nieces from the country.

If Dr Cassidy and Arthur Ward were the joint foci of the Doctor's life at St Thomas's, they were a long way from filling it. The rest of the time was devoted to surgery and an assortment of special subjects. For surgery, in which theatre lists might go on until 7 p.m., he was attached to Max, later Sir Max, Page's firm. Page, large and bluff and handsome, was a delightful man, but it became increasingly evident to the Doctor that he was not a surgeon in bud. The most vivid impression the Doctor retained from the theatre sessions was of the beauty of women's eyes. Seen above a mask they were spell-binding. When the mask was removed the revelation could be cruelly disappointing.

Surgical theory was learned from a text book which had a 'house flavour', since its authors, Mitchiner and Romanis, were both Thomas's men. Philip Mitchiner was the most colourful and unorthodox person then on the staff. An immensely able surgeon, he was reputed not to have cost his parents a penny since the age of eleven, having won every prize and scholarship open to him since that time. He wore his hair en brosse, which was unusual for the period, and did not run a car, relying on his feet or taxis, and was given to making deliberately shocking statements in a voice whose cadences were themselves shocking in a place which echoed with flawlessly U accents. The violent tongue and unconventional manner went with the kindest heart in the hospital. During the First World War Mitchiner had served as an Army surgeon in Serbia. During the Second, he was called up as a brigadier and sent to Norway, where he earned much kudos, when his unit was retreating down a road under shellfire, by walking while the others ran. Later he told the Doctor, whose patient he had become, that he had already started to suffer from angina, and was much more afraid of provoking an attack by hurrying than he was of the shells.

Special subjects, skins and chests and VD, eyes and orthopaedics and ENT, had to be fitted in as and how one could manage them. The Doctor found above his head a good deal of the teaching on eyes, but he had to admit to a lack of enthusiasm about the subject. ENT was dull when you had to be lucky to get a squint up a nostril or down an ear, and he was not greatly interested in surgery anyway. Skins were offputting because of the outlandish terminology involved: not until he was in practice did the Doctor realise what a large part they played in the work of a GP. Chests, essentially, meant TB, which, forty years ago, was a scourge against which there was no protection and for which there was no effective remedy. The best that could be hoped for was that a period in a sanatorium might restore the patient to a state in which, even if he lived to the normal span, he would be lucky indeed if he were able to lead a fully active life. Nor, even in a medical setting, could one rely on the early diagnosis which improved the chances of recovery. One day the Doctor and a fellow student, who had been a contemporary at Cambridge, were testing each other's vital capacities. The Doctor pumped out the six litres of breath which was about the norm for a healthy young man; his partner barely managed three and a half. He was known to have had pleurisy but he had not been given an X-ray and TB was not diagnosed until the time when he was qualifying. He lived only another two years.

Some other subjects were rather a joke. One learned to dispense, and make pills and wrap up medicine bottles, but none of it was very serious. The public vaccinator, who had side-whiskers and a box hat, came in an old-fashioned cape and an old-fashioned car to demonstrate his art. In vacuo, like that, it was boring. The way to learn to vaccinate, as the Doctor was later to discover, is to have to vaccinate 200-300 people at a sitting.

Infectious diseases required the students, robed in white gowns, to put in six attendances at the Western Fever Hospital, Seagrove Road, where Dr J.D. Rolleston presided. His brother, Sir Humphrey Rolleston, Regius Professor of Physick, had been a fellow-student with the Doctor's father at St George's which had brought his son occasional invitations to tea or luncheon when he was at the university. Dr Rolleston was an ardent classicist who dwelled upon the way fevers had been described by the ancients. Try as he might, the Doctor could not beat up much interest in scarlet fever according to Herodotus, or whoever. Also, he found it distressing that children who came into the Western Fever with one infection were quite likely to pick up another one or two while they were there, so that their stay might lengthen from weeks to months, during which time they got no education. But he perked up when Dr Rolleston told the students that diphtheria had a characteristic smell which, once identified, they would never mistake. That was a piece of useful, practical knowledge. The

Doctor sniffed like a trailhound until he was certain that he would be able to identify the smell anywhere. It was not to be so long before he had the opportunity.

For 'loonies' you went to Bedlam on six successive Saturday mornings – at that time the Bethlem Royal Hospital was still in the building now occupied by the Imperial War Museum. Students were apt to regard the elderly physician who conducted these sessions as something of a joke. The Doctor found the visits rather unpleasant. You had no personal contact with the patients, they were just demonstrated; and he felt a mixture of shyness and revulsion as one after another was presented. They did not seem to mind, but how could you really tell? Fortunately he had not been long at St Thomas's before the alienist retired, to be succeeded by Dr Henry Yellowlees, who brought a great light and created an interest where, before, there had been none.

Gynaecology and midwifery, thanks largely to A.J. Wrigley, were fascinating from the outset. Wrigley, the Obstetrical and Gynaecological Registrar, who was a Northerner, was a brilliant teacher who opened up the subject for the benefit of all. Dr Bamforth, a pathologist, who worked closely with him, was also from the North. He was a Liverpudlian, clever, single-minded and down-to-earth, whose lectures were liable to contain imperishable phrases like the description of a specimen as having 'a moth-eaten appearance, as though nibbled by a mouse'. Already he was doing cervical smears for the early detection of cancer.

It was 'midder' that gave you your first taste of being on your own. Each student had to look after twenty confinements before his Finals. The job was learned on half a dozen in the Maternity Ward, where delivery was done by Sister or Staff Nurse, with a doctor, House Physician, Registrar or First Assistant, on tap in case of difficulties. After that the students, working in pairs, were sent out on to the district, which then included part of Lewisham and the Elephant, as well as Lambeth. For a month at a time successive groups of eight students moved into 'midder digs' in the area surrounding the hospital, Lambeth Palace Road, Paris Street, Paradise Street, chosen so that the hospital porter could knock them up for night calls. It was the first time the Doctor had left Queen's Gate Gardens; he enjoyed the liberty even if the food was a bit of a come-down.

Around 1930 the district patients were not among the tele-phone subscribing classes. Some member of the family, on foot or bicycle, was sent posting off to the hospital when the mother went into labour, and the lodge porter detained the messenger to act as guide while he alerted the pair of students who were next on the list. A 'gamp', a sort of home help, who saw that hot water was available, and tidied up generally, was allotted to each case, but the two students looked after the delivery.

Now you began to feel some responsibility; though you could send to the hospital for help if you were in trouble, there were some emergencies which you just had to get on with by yourself. The question of judgment came into it, too. If you sent for help unnecessarily you got a rocket, but it was nothing like the one you got if you did not send when you should have done. In twelve hours you came back, and again on the follow-ing day, then over the next ten days you would visit like a GP. Since you would probably have two or three cases to look after, it was quite possible that you might be up most of the night, have to visit during the day, then be up again during the next night. By the end of the month you were quite tired. But at least you had nothing else to do during the month, except keep your 'midder' bag up to date, and attend Joe Wrigley's classes, and get down to your books between calls. The Doctor feels sorry for today's students, because they have so much theory to absorb. In his day, when there were virtually no treatments, there was correspondingly less chemical detail which had to be learned.

'Major week' was another endurance test, if a less taxing one. Its setting was Night Casualty, where four medical and four surgical firms took turns to receive patients in Casualty, and the pair of students on duty spent the night in the little 'major-week' dressers' room. From 7 p.m. to midnight or 1 a.m. things would be pretty brisk; after that you would get a chance to lie down – probably to be called up again. It was here that one picked up tips which were to be invaluable in practice and were useful on the spot – the price of failing to plug a bleeding tooth socket effectively, for instance, was to be called up again. You followed through the cases you admitted, but you worked under the supervision of a qualified doctor.

31

All the surgical emergencies were seen by the Resident Assistant Surgeon, who operated intermittently from 8 p.m. to 1 or 2 a.m. When he had a night off, the Surgical Registrar, who normally lived out, came in to replace him.

Not until about the time the Doctor was qualifying did higher authority realise that the two Residents, Physician and Surgeon, were grossly overworked, and appoint extra Registrars to every firm and to the special departments. The immediate consequence was alarm and despondency among the housemen, who feared that their work would be taken from them, but there turned out to be enough for all, and besides the Registrars went home at night.

'Major week' revealed to the Doctor the seamy side of Lambeth and Lewisham. People who came into Casualty at night were really ill, or severely injured or very drunk indeed. The atmosphere was more dramatic than by day, with attendant crowds of weeping relatives to point the occasional tragedies. It made curiously little impression on a young man who had, perhaps, a rather larger allowance of compassion in his make-up than the average, and whose life hitherto had certainly not been a toughening course. Partly it was because he was there to do something about the situation, not to indulge in the luxury of private feelings; more, he realised later, it was the result of the hospital situation, in which doctor and patient played their ceremonial roles, the former knowing nothing of the past or future of the people he treated. Detachment was to be less easy for a GP who was personally involved in the home background of his patients.

Inevitably, the teaching was variable, but, looking back, the Doctor rates the general level as very high. There were negative lessons as well as positive; some subjects were neglected or looked down on, and some were not taught at all. Well before he was ready to qualify, the Doctor had had from certain of the 'honoraries' demonstrations of how one should not as well as how one should interview patients. Teachers may have dropped hints on patient handling, but if so they were so well concealed among clinical detail that it was fairly easy to miss them. Only the paediatrician made any attempt to separate the technical from the human side of his cases – it was vitally necessary to do so when dealing with children. Even at that stage the Doctor felt that it was a pity more adults were not treated like children.

Years later, when he learned of Sir James Spence's work at Newcastle-on-Tyne, he envied retrospectively the students who, during outpatient clinics, were taught, not the techniques of diagnosis and treatment, which, of course, had their place elsewhere in the curriculum, but the art of consultation. And he would have underwritten Spence's dictum that 'the real work of a doctor' and 'the essential unit of medical practice' is that intimate, person-to-person contact between practitioner and patient which takes place in the surgery. He noted, too, that once more it was a paediatrician who was proclaiming that principle – Sir James Spence was the first whole-time Professor of Child Health in Britain.

Industrial medicine cropped up only incidentally, in relation to particular cases of 'barman's TB', or oil dermatitis, or silicosis in miners. There was no teaching about psychosomatic illness as such, though that, too, sometimes came up in individual cases because a number of physicians were aware of it. The Doctor himself recognised comparatively early on the part played by the emotions in physical disease, but he realised that the help a doctor could give was limited when he did not know or understand the patient's home environment. Neither did social medicine exist as a subject, though it was almost impossible to avoid some reference to it. Nonetheless, some surgeons, and even some physicians, managed to do so.

In theory public health had a place in the curriculum; in practice it was openly despised by teachers and gladly neglected by students. The reasons for the attitude of the teachers were partly personal, partly historical. They themselves were interested almost exclusively in the pathology of disease, and the idea had survived from another age that public health was a matter of drains and water supplies, and since both were now reliable in Britain, there was no longer any need to bother about it. The MOH was considered inferior: students learned that they must get in touch with him if they happened on a case of smallpox, but were given no idea of the close connection which should exist between GP and local authority. Indeed, though the great majority of them intended to be GPs, they got no teaching whatever about the running of a practice, whether from the point of view of economics or the point of view of administration. You picked up what you could from contemporaries whose fathers were GPs, or from meeting former students now in practice.

Even with so many omissions, it was a full programme, and private life was virtually relegated to the week-ends. The Doctor had picked up again the friendship with one of his earliest schoolfellows, who had shared the wonder of Mrs Chitty's demonstrating how the world revolved on its axis, whose family had recently returned to Slough after some years' absence. In contrast to his own home, which, with his sister away and his brother spending much of his leisure playing golf, was a little quiet and lonely, their house seemed always full of talk, and music, and young people. He spent most of his time there, and became increasingly drawn to his friend's younger sister. They became engaged just after he had done his 'midder' – did all those babies make him go broody? – in the resigned knowledge that it would be an awfully long engagement. You didn't get married until you could support a wife. Relatively speaking, his fiancée was a woman of substance, because she earned between £2 and £3 a week by working for a cousin who ran a dress shop in Beauchamp Place, but at least he was in a position to drive her home for the week-end and bring her back to London. At that period the alternative was a two-and-sixpenny return ticket on the Green Line, or the Premier Service, which, in winter, provided rugs for its passengers.

For the other five days of the week the Doctor was part of the hospital as one is part of a regiment or a ship's company, leaving it in the evenings for dinner, only to get down to work afterwards. He had not been persuaded to join any of the various student societies; he had had to give up rowing during his last year at Cambridge, because of a hernia, the sequel, undoubtedly, of the operations of his schooldays. The damage had been repaired, of course, but even if it had been wise to start rowing again, the tideway was profoundly uninviting after the river. So he spent every available moment of the day watching and listening and asking questions. The old Cambridge habit of tea and gossip in the club at the end of the day, followed by an hour or two of bridge for relaxation, persisted, but the gossip, now, was shop talk, and this was not Cambridge. The atmosphere of the hospital, indeed, was strikingly different from that of the university. At that time it was still

34

possible to take eight or ten years over qualifying, in contrast to the present day, when more than one examination failure means the withdrawal of a local authority grant, but not many, in fact, did so. This was a place where people had come to learn their trade, and you sensed it. The students were older, politics were more evident than they had been at Cambridge, with the House of Commons across the river as a symbol. There was even one student who marched with Mosley. He was considered a queer fish, but so long as he did not wear his black shirt in the hospital, which would not have gone down at all well, nobody minded what he did in his free time. Straining charity, somebody even suggested that, as he was interested in psychology, he might have been studying human reaction in crowds.

The biggest difference was that St Thomas's, standing at the dead centre of London, with trams, and Foden steam waggons, and horse-drawn drays with solid tyres rattling and clattering past it all day long, and pile drivers working on Lambeth Bridge, was in the world as the landlocked peace of a Cambridge college could never be. The world flowed through its doors. Occasionally the hospital impinged upon the world in unexpected ways, as on the day when a tram, lurching along Lambeth Palace Road, shaved a passing horse and cart and ripped open the horse's jugular vein. The dramatic gush of blood would have meant the end of the poor beast long before a veterinary surgeon could have reached the spot, but Dr Hector Goadby, Resident Assistant Physician, happened to be crossing the road at that moment and to have an arterial clamp in his pocket. He paused long enough to apply it, and the horse lived to pull another dray.

At the same time the hospital was a world of its own, a close community of skill and suffering and work and devotion and discipline, in which young men brought suddenly face to face with the fundamentals of life and death found relief in the normal amount of bawdy and spasmodic rowdyism. Some of the lighter flights were quite gay. There was a morning when a battered, deplorably non-vintage car, labelled: 'The carriage which was driven by Sir Percy Sargent (then Senior Surgeon) round the field of Waterloo', appeared in the Central Hall, just round the corner from the bay in the corridor where was displayed as an object of veneration the carriage in which Florence Nightingale, founder of the Nurses' Training School which bears her name, drove round the Crimea. Miss Lloyd Still was not amused. The crocodile of fledgling Nightingales from the Preliminary Training School who, led by Home Sister, were daily marched along the corridor on the way to lunch, were on that day warned before they set out that they were not, repeat *not*, to look to their left as they passed through the Hall, though they were not told what it was they must not see. God is not mocked. . . .

CHAPTER 3

QUALIFICATION:
DOCTOR IN THE HOUSE

He qualified in the summer of 1930, at the second attempt. There was no almighty binge, just a celebration luncheon with his fiancée, in a daze of relief. There had been so many times when he felt he would never get to the end of what seemed the interminable road ahead. True, there was his Cambridge examination to take again, because he had failed that also at the first go, and he was twenty-five and so far had not earned a penny, and heaven knew how many more years it would be before he could get married, but, for the moment, none of that mattered! He was a doctor. As soon as he knew the result he had gone straight from Queen's Square to the offices of the Medical Defence Union to take out the insurance against the hideous possibility of claims from dissatisfied patients; such insurance cover was a necessity, or at least a highly desirable precaution, for every doctor. Then he sat down to consider the realities.

At that time it was not compulsory, as it is today, to spend twelve months in junior hospital posts between qualifying and entering practice. With the 'conjoint' in his pocket, the Doctor, like the rest of his newly fledged colleagues, was entitled to start directly in practice. Perhaps more from enlightened self-interest than from a sense of responsibility towards their future patients, few of them did so; and virtually none went into single-handed practice, where they realised that their lack of experience would be highly likely to lead to financial failure if not more dramatic disaster.

The norm after qualification was to serve in junior house appointments, which gave them further experience in general medicine and in subjects that are of major importance in family practice: paediatrics, or child health, and obstetrics and gynaecology. In the teaching hospitals these posts were unpaid. In other hospitals, in various parts of the country, rates varied from £25 to £75 for six months' work. On an average, the young doctors spent two to two-and-a-half years in this way, though there were a few who entered practice as assistants or very junior partners after a shorter period.

The nature and conditions of that voluntarily undertaken period of further training make an interesting comparison with the various schemes for vocational training for general practitioners which have developed in recent years. Typically, they last three years; one year is spent in practice under a GP who undertakes the responsibility of teaching and supervising the trainee, and two years are spent in hospital posts. Paediatrics, obstetrics and gynaecology figure largely in the hospital posts, and there are shorter attachments to departments such as Casualty, Ophthalmology, Dermatology and Ear, Nose and Throat. Two subjects which often appear in today's courses would not have been considered worth the attention of an aspiring GP in the early 1930s; they are geriatrics, or the medicine of old age, and psychiatry. Trainees are paid – or were paid at the time of writing – a little over £2,000 a year. According to a report in the *British Medical Journal* on the training scheme in Newcastle-on-Tyne, some complained of the financial loss they incurred. Three years of vocational training would leave them worse off by £5,030 than their colleagues who had entered partnership at the end of their compulsory twelve months' hospital service, with no further training; and they suggested that, on completing the three years, they should receive this sum as a bonus.

It was usual to put in for house appointments at one's own hospital, since holding a job at it was equivalent to getting one's First Eleven colours, but competition was keen, and less than half of those who qualified each year could be successful. Eight new young doctors were appointed as Casualty Officers every six months, at the end of which time half went on to be House Surgeons, half to be House Physicians. Besides those appointments, there were about eighteen jobs in specialist departments, which were held for six months, and which were not preceded by a term as Casualty Officer. The Doctor would have taken anything that offered, but, hopefully, he put in an application for Casualty Officer and House Physician. Qualifying as he had in June, he could not get a house appointment of any kind until the end of the year. He wanted a holiday, he wanted some money and he wanted to fill the waiting time usefully.

The last problem was solved by his getting a Clinical Assistantship in Outpatients, to be taken up in the autumn. It was, of course, unpaid, and it carried no real responsibility – that word again – but it would keep him in touch. Then came two successive strokes of luck. The first was a tutoring job which took him for a month to the West of Ireland. It involved being less a schoolmaster than a companion to a ten-year-old boy who had no contemporaries in the assembled house party. After two hours' nominal lessons each morning they had the freedom of the wild country of Connemara, so much a fisherman's paradise that you might take two sea trout on a single cast, one on the tail fly and one on the drop. At Renvyle House, near by, which had been rebuilt as a hotel after being gutted during the troubles, Augustus John was installed with his family.

During Horse Show week the entire household moved up to Dublin, where its members were put up by various friends of the family. The Doctor's host was Joyce's 'stately, plump, Buck Mulligan', Oliver St John Gogarty, poet, Senator, ear, nose and throat specialist, to adopt what would probably have been his own preferred order of precedence. It was only to be expected that he should be a brilliant conversationalist; but the Doctor was more surprised that Gogarty should get him up before breakfast to go swimming in the Dublin baths. A Corporation car and chauffeur called to drive them there and take them home again. Altogether it was so good a holiday that it seemed unbelievable to receive four guineas a week for enjoying it. Into the bargain, his charge was a likeable small boy and the Doctor got on so well with the family that, during the following summer, he was invited to join the house party as a guest.

The second piece of good fortune, coming almost immediately after his return to London, gave him his first taste of real general practice. A fellow student, son of a West Country GP, had come up to St Thomas's with the parental injunction to 'have a good time, and play some rugger, then, after you qualify, you can join me here and take over when I finish'. He had acted on the first part of it so enthusiastically that he was not within hailing distance of qualification when his father developed heart trouble and it became evident that the time-table would have to be speeded up. The son got down to work while, to bridge the gap, a succession of his newly qualified contemporaries, the Doctor among them, went down for a few weeks at a time to act as assistant in his father's practice.

On paper the situation might have seemed dismaying for a young man fresh from a top teaching hospital, just as a fishing village in remote North Devon might have seemed primitive after the well-groomed Home Counties. Dr Vere ran a single-handed practice in a one-doctor district which covered the whole village and part of a neighbouring small town. He was a widower, looked after by a housekeeper, his surgery and waiting-room were pretty gloomy, and he did his rounds in an elderly Ford. In fact, at that period, young men from London had great respect for a doctor who was doing a good job in conditions which, inevitably, were those of a cottage industry, and they regarded as a stimulating challenge the opportunity of working among a population which, because of its relative remoteness from any large town, had had less intensive doctoring than a comparable urban community.

The Doctor knew that he had everything to learn about general practice, and recognised from the start that Dr Vere, old and wise and easy-going, and a jolly good doctor, was an excellent person to teach him. He spent the day visiting on foot, while his senior did a morning round of private patients in the Ford and rested in the afternoons. The Doctor found village life fascinating and got on well with the patients, whom he saw both in their homes and at the evening panel surgery. Dr Vere explained how the panel worked, and, since the token pharmacy imparted at St Thomas's was already forgotten, taught him how to dispense and wrap bottles. More important, he trusted the young man, was ready to discuss cases with him, and, over meals and during evenings spent in the first-floor sitting-room, dipped into a store of anecdotes accumulated over forty years of practice in country and small town interspersed with a period of service in Serbia during the First World War, during part of which he had been physician to the unit of which Philip Mitchiner was surgeon.

The anecdotes did not lack drama. There were apt to be extraordinary emergencies, for it was the period when there

40

were no medical benefits, and patients who were at once stoical and thrifty got into remarkable states. When a little girl came pelting into the surgery crying: 'Doctor, doctor, come quick! Grannie's gallstones is rattling down the stairs!' they really were, from a ruptured gall bladder. For the Doctor the generality of the practice was typified by a chair which Dr Vere had in his surgery. It had come from a ship which was being broken up at a yard near by, and it was part operating table, part dental chair. It would immobilise a patient and, in the rather remote event of its being necessary, crucify him.

Dr Vere was a father figure to the village – sometimes a rather fierce one. Once he told the young assistant that if ever any cases of VD cropped up he made sure the victims were 'sent away' to prevent its spreading, but he did not explain how this was done, so one had to take his word for it.

Dr Vere recalled that once, while he and the local midwife were waiting for a baby to arrive, he had asked: 'Kate, when do the boys and girls start going together?' and Kate had replied: 'Oh, before they leave school.' The young assistant took that early indication of a permissive society in his stride. One accepted that, in the country, pregnancy often preceded marriage, being regarded as evidence that a young woman was fitted for it. By contrast, he found himself rather upset when, as he was on a Sunday morning round, he met, drifting down the street in beach pyjamas, with a long cigarette holder, one of the Society celebrities of the day stoned cold. He knew, of course, if only in theory, that such things happened in London, but they seemed worse in a village, with the sea at the end of the street, and the women standing at their gates, knitting. They wore a belt with a protective leather pad slung over their left hip, with the left hand resting against it, holding one knitting needle immobile; while the right hand worked at such speed that a jersey would be completed in three days.

Those six weeks confirmed the Doctor in his decision that, wherever he did it, general practice was what he wanted to do. It had been a valuable as well as a fascinating experience, and he had even earned some money. After so many years he cannot remember whether his salary was six or seven guineas a week, all found: either way it was wealth compared with what had gone before and what was to come after. What came immediately afterwards was the Clinical Assistantship in Outpatients, which filled in the time until the New Year, when he became a Casualty Officer. The eight newly qualified doctors serving the department were supervised by a senior who had himself spent six months as a Casualty Officer and done one, perhaps two, house jobs before being appointed to the senior post for a year. Each ran his own clinic, with the help of a group of students, and also acted as resident anaesthetist – training in anaesthetics, given by the 'honoraries', was included in the surgical part of the students' course. Acting as resident anaesthetist involved going to any department where one might be needed. Mostly it was to fill gaps, since the bulk of the work was done by the honorary anaesthetists appointed to the hospital, but the young residents might get the unimportant cases at the end of the list. Once he had got the hang of it, which he did rather quickly, the Doctor enjoyed this more than any other part of the casualty job. It was new to be left alone with patients, and he found it satisfying. With luck you got a bite of supper after the end of the day's lists, before starting to give anaesthetics for the Resident Assistant Surgeon who had to deal with the surgical emergencies which came in a steady stream after 7 p.m. In a desultory fashion these evening sessions might go on until midnight, and after that you were liable to be fetched out of bed. Every other evening you got off between 7 and 8 p.m., and, barring emergencies, alternate week-ends were free.

The Casualty Officers had bed-sitters in the students' club over the way, and fed in College House, a block in the hospital which contained living quarters for the House Physicians and Surgeons who had to be on the spot. It was back to school or university. The dining-room had a board floor and, above a dark green dado, dingy cream walls lined with groups of College House fifty years ago. The two shabby leather club armchairs were the only easy chairs available to junior staff, except for the one which each had in his bed-sitter. Again as at school, meals were ample and solid and low in Vitamin C. In winter one sometimes got a salad of endive, but the vegetables were boiled to battered wedges of cellulose, and there was scarcely any fresh fruit. If there could be said to be a *spécialité de la maison* it was the apple dumplings. They were huge, made from full-sized Bramleys. Johnnie Johnstone, who had an enormous mouth, was once bet five bob that he wouldn't get a whole one in without spluttering bits out. He won. Just.

The Casualty Officers and young housemen got no pay, unless you counted the half-pint of light beer that went with lunch and supper. Your salary was your board and lodging, and you paid for your own washing.

To the Doctor's knowledge only one of his contemporaries was married – well, how could you be on two bottles of beer a day? – and he had been married as a student. Accordingly, there was no demand for married quarters. Neither did anybody feel he was being victimised. All the residents were doing a job they had wanted to do, in appointments which they had been delighted to get, and which were recognised as being the best way to start a career. Their aim, now, was to get as much experience as possible. A day of at least twelve hours was considered normal. Small perks like the two guineas received for making a report on injuries to enable a patient to make an insurance or compensation claim, or the shilling for every infectious fever notified, were gratefully received, but, over the six months of their appointments, would not have amounted to more than £5 to £10 for house physicians and perhaps £20 for house surgeons.

What were the criteria of the medical committee in making appointments to house jobs, given the obvious condition that they had to choose from what was offered? Prizemen were likely to get the best jobs, but being good at exams did not seem to have much to do with it. The committee knew that the Doctor was a bad exam passer, that he had entered the Medical School without a Second MB, that he had had one failure in his Cambridge examination and that he had only the 'conjoint'. Was there an element of nepotism? Could the fact that he had had a personal introduction to Dr Cassidy have led to the Doctor's appointment as his House Physician? He would very much like to think that it did not, but to this day he does not seem quite certain.

At the time he had no thought to spare for such scruples. This was the job for which he had longed since first he became a medical student. At last he had responsibility for the management of forty-five patients.

Forty years ago the pattern of illness was in many ways different from that of today: for a generation which has grown up to take antibiotics for granted, the situation is difficult to envisage. Since there was no reliable method of dealing with acute infection, pneumonia, for instance, had to be allowed to run its course, whether that course led to the dramatic crisis of lobar pneumonia, so beloved of Victorian novelists, or was the long-drawn-out one of the commoner broncho-pneumonia. Broncho-pneumonia was often nursed at home; if the patient was of sufficient distinction, straw was laid over the road outside to muffle the noise of horse-drawn traffic, clopping hoofs and iron-rimmed wheels. There were also, forty years ago, more young people in hospital with heart conditions following rheumatic fever, which was still relatively common compared with the present day, when streptococcal infection has been almost defeated. There was little that could be done for them except hope that, with adequate rest, the heart might build up some reserve.

Pernicious anaemia was still a killer, though not an immediate one: sufferers had recurrent attacks, with remissions, over anything from two to five years. It had recently been discovered that patients fed on raw liver improved, but if they were to survive, they were faced with the necessity of getting down a pound of it every day for the rest of their lives. The break-through in this lay in the near future. First, a liver extract, which had the same effect and which could be injected, was produced; then it was found that the vital principle was Vitamin B 12, which need be given only about once a month. To this day there is still no cure for pernicious anaemia: it can only be controlled, like diabetes. The latter had been controllable for the past ten years or so, but there was still no prolonged-action insulin.

Anti-tetanus serum had been in use for some time. A very recent development was the anti-serum used in desperate cases of streptococcal pneumonia. Desperate cases only, because the allergic reactions could be almost as bad as the original disease; sometimes, indeed, fatal. Today the pneumonia would have been treated early with appropriate antibiotics.

In the early 1930s St Thomas's was admitting a certain number of cases of GPI (general paralysis of the insane) which were the legacy of syphylis contracted ten or twenty years earlier, possibly during the First World War. Cure there was none: treatments, some of which had a certain effect, were many. It had been noticed that patients who had suffered a high temperature improved, so this was produced artificially. One method was to give the GPI patient two or three times the normal dose of typhoid vaccine, which sent his temperature up to 103 or 104, and repeat the process every two or three days over a fortnight. At St Thomas's, when the Doctor took up his appointment as House Physician, it was done by giving them malaria. A man from the Ministry of Health arrived with a muslin cage of malaria-carrying mosquitoes which was strapped to the leg of the patient until its inmates were gorged. About a fortnight later his temperature would show the alternate rise and fall of malaria. When it was considered that the process had lasted long enough, the malaria was treated with quinine. The patients did indeed show an improvement. The Doctor suspected that the situation deteriorated rather soon, though he was never able to follow up a case.

But then, house officers, holding their appointments for six months, seldom did see their patients after they had been discharged, and so were spared the knowledge of how soon some of them went downhill after they had returned to the conditions of wretched housing and exiguous feeding which had helped to bring them to hospital in the first place.

The Doctor never had any difficulty in getting on with his patients, and developed a fairly close relationship with those who remained in hospital for many weeks. Later, he came to realise that, despite good will on both sides, it had been a rather formal relationship, not to be compared with that which a GP develops with his patients, and to understand that it could hardly have been otherwise in a situation in which both sides were out of their natural element. In the hospital ward the patient was cast to express the quality of gratitude, the doctor that of magnanimity: the atmosphere had nothing to do with the former and not a great deal to do with the latter; its focus was the fact of disease.

At the time the doctor was only dimly, if at all, aware of these things, and the days were too full and too absorbing to allow leisure for brooding over them. Every morning he did a ward round with Sister, examining patients and ordering the necessary investigations. It was a feather in your cap if you managed to get them all done before the 'honorary's' first

45

round after the patients had been admitted, but it took determined beavering to achieve that. Things like blood counts and blood sugar the Doctor did himself in the labs available. It was possible to get investigations done in the official labs, but if you overburdened them with simple things they were apt to grumble and send them back. That kind of work had to be fitted into the evenings, since the days were spent chiefly on the ward. In the evenings, also, he sometimes did minor operations like tapping a chest to draw off fluid, or opening an abscess. About 10 p.m. there was a night round to make sure that all was well, and there were notes of patients due for discharge to be written up. There was no routine about letters to GPs. There were no secretaries either. It was left to the House Physician to give the GP a précis of his patient's case and indicate whether he still needed to be on active treatment, and he did so in his own longhand. If the house physician was lazy or did not think it necessary, there was no letter. The process worked the other way, also. So scrappy, cursory and even downright inaccurate were some of the 'letters' which certain GPs gave to patients whom they were referring to hospital that the Doctor took a vow that, when he himself was in practice, he would never send one of his patients to hospital without a properly informative letter.

In between all that, one tried to find time for some professional reading. Not surprisingly, the Doctor was able to do very little, but, none the less, when he went up for a second go at his Cambridge exam, he passed it rather easily. Dealing with patients had given him the confidence he had previously lacked. The only hitch, and that a minor one, concerned photographs of children with malformations. He failed to recognise malformation due to rickets, but the examiner, a slim, lively senior physician with a carnation in his buttonhole, was very nice about it, since, as he said, one did not see rickets these days. 'Oh, yes you do', said the Doctor. The examiner was unconvinced, the candidate polite but obdurate. A few months later, when the candidate was House Physician at the Victoria Hospital for Children in Tite Street, Chelsea, he took quiet pleasure in admitting six children from the same family, all with marked rachitic deformities, to that senior physician's beds on the same day. Dr Douglas Firth took it very well. Later, his wife and daughters were to be the

Doctor's patients as long as they remained in the area.

From his first days in the hospital the Doctor had admired the ward sisters at St Thomas's, but it was during his period as House Physician that he came fully to realise their worth. It was inestimable. He himself was now personally involved with the problems of his patients in a way that he had not been as a student, but often they wanted to talk to an older person rather than to a very young doctor, and the older person was usually Sister. House Physicians changed every six months, 'Honoraries' appeared on two afternoons a week. Sister, in those days, stayed for five, or ten, or even twenty years. She ensured continuity in the ward situation, and, very largely, it was she who saw that standards were maintained. Young housemen were sometimes pretty inept at first. Sister, if she was tactful, could provide unobtrusive guidance, leading from behind and sometimes steering them away from potential trouble. But if there had ever been a head-on confrontation between Sister and young doctor where the welfare of a patient was at stake, there was little room to doubt who would have won. Along with the skill, and the dedication, and the almost invariable piety, there was an element of steel in the heiresses and guardians of Miss Nightingale's tradition.

The young Doctor's day, which had started with a morning round with Sister, ended somewhere about midnight, when the lamp at the nurse's station in the centre of each ward was shaded, and crickets chirped in the lifts – after the war they had vanished; was it DDT or just attrition? – and the Casualty Officer or House Physician, moving about the darkened Central Hall building, would cross Night Sister on her rounds. Night Sister of that period had a miraculous faculty of being all over the hospital all the time, materialising instantly at moments of crisis. Like all Night Sisters, she never passed along the central corridor without an automatic glance at the statue of the Founder of the Nightingale School of Nursing. Periodically, graceless students crowned it with a chamber pot, and it was one of the unofficial duties of Night Sisters to get a step ladder and remove the article before dawn and the coming of Matron. There was a night, too, when the busts of the founding fathers of medicine which adorned the Central Hall were changed round. One was even placed in Matron's office, which, in theory, was securely locked against intruders.

To this day there is said to be no certainty that all the heads are back on the right plinths.

Night Sister was known also for somehow finding time to chase young residents who looked as if they were starting 'flu or running a temperature, getting them into a mustard bath and following up with heroic doses of whisky from the ward medicine chest. She was later heard of at Dunkirk, administering brandy gargles to the troops and telling them to swallow. It was absolutely in character, the Doctor reflected when he heard that story, and it would have been neat brandy, too. It was doubtful if Night Sister herself had ever tasted anything stronger than dry sherry, unlike Sister City, a remarkable character who ran a small antique business in her sitting-room and was reputed to enjoy her glass.

When the twelve months of jobs at St Thomas's ended, the Doctor went on to be resident house physician at the Victoria Hospital for Children, armed with Dr Cassidy's reference. If there had been a touch of nepotism about his appointment, at least the boss did not seem to have found any reason to regret it. The scrawled paper said just: 'The best House Physician I have ever had'.

The Doctor's arrival at Tite Street was traumatic. A pretty and amiable Sister met him at the door of the ground floor medical ward to accompany him on his first round, but he was scarcely over the threshold when he froze like a pointer. There, unmistakably, was the smell which, during his student visits to the Western Fever Hospital, he had learned to recognise as characteristic of diphtheria, which Dr Rolleston had said could never be missed once it had been identified. Despite his horror some instinct counselled caution. 'Sister,' he said tentatively, 'what is this smell? It seems familiar, but I can't quite place it.' 'Oh,' replied Sister, 'you mean the oil of sassafras.' At a time when large numbers of children had infested heads, all were given the standard treatment as a matter of course when they were admitted to hospital. The Doctor never did learn the smell of diphtheria.

His two resident jobs at St Thomas's had provided wonderful experience, but, for a future GP, the six months at Tite Street, for which he was paid £50, was the most valuable part of his training. In a smaller hospital you got a wider picture than was possible in a big one, where you were limited to your own group. Consultants from a number of teaching hospitals came to work there, which broadened one's ideas and approach; GPs often came to watch operations on small patients who had been admitted to the private wing, and there would be talk about various aspects of practice.

Dr Jewesbury, the children's physician, who was an 'Honorary' at St Thomas's, was a Truby King enthusiast, so, willy nilly, one learned a good deal about that method of child care. Dr Neil Hobhouse, the neurologist, a former Thomas's student, who was at that time on the staff of the Royal Free Hospital, was particularly interested in spastic children, so there were quite a few of them in the wards for remedial exercises and physiotherapy. Dr Stanley Wyard, the pathologist, spent a good part of every day in the laboratory; you could go and ask him questions and discuss cases. Dr Douglas Firth, of the Cambridge viva, bore no malice about the rickets and advised the Doctor on the thesis which he had to produce to finalise his MB. He wrote on chronic chests – Tite Street in those days had its quota of poorly nourished children who stayed in hospital for two or more months with chest infections that would not clear up – and supported it with X-ray pictures. The thesis was accepted and the Doctor felt confident that, had he been staying on at Tite Street as Resident Medical Officer, or Registrar, he would have had no difficulty in improving it to the standard of an MD thesis. Fresh experiences included also his first acquaintance with a female doctor, though he had, of course, encountered women medical students at Cambridge. His opposite number, the House Surgeon, was an efficient young woman, the daughter of a well-known surgeon. They got on agreeably enough on the basis of neither being wildly attracted by the other: it occurred to the Doctor that, had there been a serious emotional interest, the situation might have become intolerable.

Tite Street, too, had a Casualty department, where the Doctor spent three mornings a week. It was there that he learned to examine an ear, for there was more earache than almost anything else. When one found the drum to be red and bulging, it was the signal for the operation of myringotomy, the insertion of a small knife to let out the pus, which otherwise, as the pressure built up would be forced into the air cells of the mastoid process. When that happened there was a

49

serious risk that the infection might spread inside the skull, causing an infection which could be fatal. From five to seven operations for mastoid were performed every week, Today, when antibiotics attack the infection at an early stage, myringotomy and mastoid operations are both relatively rare.

Osteomyelitis – infection of the bone – is another disease whose incidence has declined sharply since the advent of antibiotics. Then the only treatment was operation, which might or might not be successful, and there was a fairly severe mortality. Meningitis, particularly tuberculous meningitis, was a death sentence from which there was no reprieve. Among the sequence of tragic cases there stood out in the Doctor's memory that of a child born while its father was in a TB sanatorium. The parent improved so much that, at the end of six months, he was allowed home for a week-end visit. Within a fortnight the baby developed tuberculous meningitis; within a week of admission to Tite Street it was dead.

Twice a week a group of a dozen or so children were brought in to have their tonsils taken out by the guillotine method in the Outpatients' theatre. The guillotine, now happily, outmoded, was an instrument embodying a metal ring which went round the back of the tonsil and a blade which slid down on to the front of the root, so that, in theory, it could be neatly removed. In practice, fairly often, the root was not completely extracted, whereas it was not unknown for part of the throat to be taken out with the tonsil. The time available to the surgeon depended very largely on the skill of his anaesthetist, and anaesthesia was still in the heroic period. Ethyl chloride, which was highly volatile, was sprayed on to the mask as it lay on the table and it was then placed on the child's face. It was a dodgy process, since children who held their breath at first were liable suddenly to take a big breath, inhale a lot of vapour lying under the mask near the mouth and go into deep unconsciousness. One had to steer a delicate course between this and a state of too-light anaesthesia, from which the child might begin to come round while the operation was in progress. There was a similar performance during dental sessions, when a dozen teeth might be removed with the same anaesthetic.

Less the bloodstains, the weekly whooping cough clinic, whose patients announced themselves from afar, was almost equally harrowing. The children were often very ill, and, beyond trying to build up their general state and instruct mothers that the way to prevent the weight loss caused by vomiting was to see that a child which lost its dinner in a paroxysm of coughing got another immediately, there was little to be done. This was one disease for which antibiotics, when they came, could do nothing, though they were valuable in treating the secondary infections which almost always developed. After the war better prophylactics replaced the pre-war injections, which had little effect, but it was some years before the appearance of chloramphenicol, the one drug which had a direct effect. It had, however, to be used with extreme circumspection, because of its potentially damaging effect on the blood. Pending, there was a picturesque interlude at the end of the 1940s, when, it having been noticed that child whooping cough sufferers were improved after flight, arrangements were made for them to be taken for flips from Northolt. The good effect was supposed to be produced by the rapid reduction of atmospheric pressure as the aircraft rose, so that living at a high altitude would have been no substitute. Later, the patients were put into a decompression chamber instead of being given air trips.

Infectious diseases, at a time when the only standard protection was vaccination against smallpox, were a nightmare. Every child with a running nose had to be regarded as a diphtheria carrier, if not as a sufferer from the disease, and life was a constant round of swabbing noses and throats. Measles was dreaded above all else because it was so intensely infectious. A single case meant closing the ward to new entries for three weeks. It was possible to protect children at risk by injecting them with serum obtained by taking blood from adults who had recently had measles, but there was never enough serum available for all the children susceptible to infection; it could be obtained only for those who were already very ill with some other ailment. It occurred to the Doctor that, since most adults had had measles at some time during their lives, serum obtained from almost any adult would do as well.

When the first case of measles appeared after his appointment to Tite Street, he got in touch with all the parents of all the other children in the ward, asking them to come to the hospital, and, having established that they had had measles,

51

explained that if he could have a pint of their blood there and then he could probably prevent their child's having it. The work involved was hectic, since, to be effective, the operation had to be completed within forty-eight hours, but it came off and the ward was not closed. By the time the next measles season came round the Doctor's appointment at Tite Street had ended, so he was not able to repeat the experiment, but he did write it up for publication in one of the medical journals. To the best of his knowledge his successor did not continue the process.

Altogether, at Tite Street, even more than he had been at St Thomas's, the Doctor was in a learning situation. Most of all, the children taught him. From them he learned, among much else, that tact, kindliness, good manners and patience were essential when you were examining a child, that you should begin with the things which were the least upsetting and that you should always tell a child what you were going to do even if it could not yet talk. They taught him, too, that the proper place to examine a frightened child was on its mother's lap, and that to allow a nurse to take such a child from its mother, undress it, lay it on an examination couch and stick a thermometer up its rectum was to ensure that succeeding examinations would be a battle. Very soon the Doctor realised that time taken over a first examination would save hours in later examinations over a period of years, also that children were often as intelligent as the doctor and that it was a mistake to ignore their remarks and comments.

He could not altogether be blamed for not having learned that children up to the age of six or seven, who cannot appreciate explanations, need parental visits which are frequent and last as long as possible, for at that time almost nobody had realised that truth. Tite Street believed firmly that visits from parents upset children, and only those patients who were gravely ill might be visited on weekdays. Other children saw their parents only on Sunday afternoons, and it took the ward twenty-four hours to settle after their departure. The reason for the hospital's attitude was simple enough. At that time children who came into hospital were almost all from working-class homes, and doctors in general were not going into those homes regularly enough to see how the children reacted to hospital and how they behaved after their return home. Not until the Doctor began to pay home visits to children under the NHS did he realise how serious a degree of psychological shock they could suffer when they were suddenly deprived of the security of parental affection while still too young to understand why.

It was during his period at Tite Street that the Doctor decided that, when the time came, he would practise in London. Until then, like a good many of his contemporaries, he had had at the back of his mind the idea of a country town, perhaps in Shropshire or on the Welsh Border. It involved a Georgian house with a decent garden, perhaps a tennis court, certainly access to a trout stream. The honest work that he would put into the practice, and the responsibility entailed, would still leave leisure for the pleasures and duties that go with being a local worthy. It was a good life of its kind, and a realistic enough ambition, particularly for young men who had been to the right school and university. The two factors which led the Doctor to change his mind were his meeting with a wider range of doctors and learning from them of the possibilities in London, and the fact that his fiancée wanted to continue living there after they were married. General practice, he decided, was much the same anywhere; the obvious differences were not fundamental. The important thing was to have a happy family life.

Meantime, there was his training to finish. Upon leaving Tite Street he was reappointed to St Thomas's, successively as Gynaecological House Surgeon and Obstetrical House Physician, which meant benefiting once more from the admirable teaching of A. J. Wrigley. At the end of that year came a stroke of luck. A young doctor from the North had been appointed as Gynaecological Registrar, but before taking up the post he had to serve his terms as House Surgeon and Physician at St Thomas's, which meant that there was a six months' gap to fill. The Doctor was offered the post as a locum. It was the best job he had ever had. You were paid £5 a week, it was a non-resident and the hours were relatively easy. On the £5, with about £100 in the bank, he got married. Sister Arthur lent him her car to drive down to Devon for the honeymoon and he and his wife returned to set up house in a rented, two-room furnished flat in SW1, on a top floor with no lift.

53

As a stopgap Registrar he did not operate on his own responsibility, but he spent a good deal of time in the theatre, helped with teaching and, in the intervals, managed to work out all the statistics for the department, his predecessor having gone off to another job without ever catching up with them. At the same time he put in for an out-patient anaesthetist post which fell vacant at Tite Street, since the two sessions a week required could be fitted in with the Registrar's job. It meant a return to the fearsome tonsils and adenoids under ethyl chloride, and the money, £20 or £25 a year, was negligible, but a hospital appointment gave one a certain standing and opened the way to more private anaesthetic work. It was still the epoch when anaesthesia was largely done as a sideline by GPs. The Diploma of Anaesthesia was instituted while the Doctor held the Tite Street appointment, but though he both enjoyed the work and had an obvious flair for it, he did not feel sufficiently committed to think of taking the examination and specialising. Neither did he consider specialising in gynaecology and obstetrics.

On an income of £5 a week, life had to be pretty quiet, even though it was said at the time that it cost 15s. 0d a week to feed a man and a little less to feed a woman. But, in any case, he was so busy with the business of finding a practice to start in when the Registrar's job ended in June that there would have been little time for a full social life.

CHAPTER 4

JUNIOR PARTNER:
'GOOD FAMILY PRACTICE'

To set up in practice in the 1930s you had to have capital. For those who had none, starting as an assistant offered a side-door, but assistantships could be dicey. There was always the problem of how to stop being an assistant, since salaries were seldom large enough to offer much hope of laying aside the required amount of money to buy a share in the practice this side of one's dotage. One had to be particularly wary of assistantships 'with a view'. In theory, this meant the prospect of being offered a share in the practice at a reasonable rate at the end of six months or a year, assuming that principal and assistant were satisfied with each other. Usually, in such cases, the assistant accepted a lower salary than the norm during the probationary period. The snag was that some doctors took advantage of the opportunity of getting help on the cheap by always advertising jobs 'with a view' and never finding a candidate worthy of being offered a share.

Assuming that the young doctor, which, normally, meant his family, had some capital, the accepted ways of starting were to put up your plate or to buy a share in a practice outright, so that you entered it as a junior partner, not as an assistant. Putting up your plate was risky. It meant committing yourself to renting surgery premises and waiting for the patients to come. Success depended in about equal proportions upon the personality of the individual, the area in which he chose to start and the competition that he had to face – those who chose a district where doctors were already thick on the ground were likely to be unpopular with their colleagues – plus an element of luck.

At that time, even in London, you could rent a house for something between £120 and £400, according to size and district. Paying the rates and furnishing it would take £500 at most, another £100 would easily cover the necessary medical equipment and the essential car need not cost more than £120-£150 if you did not look higher than a Ford. For the first year you would have to live on your capital, and it would be wise not to adopt an excessively frugal life-style, since it paid to do a certain amount of entertaining and go about a bit in order to make yourself known. During the second year you would probably still be subsidising your income from capital. By the third, if you were succeeding, you should be supporting yourself and your family, provided it was not too big or too extravagant. At a pinch, £3,000 would enable you to start like that in Central London, though £4,000 would be better. If you made the grade you could expect to have an annual income of £2,000–£2,500 at the end of three years. The highly successful and fashionable might hope for a maximum of about £5,000, which meant being more than comfortably off. At the other end of the scale, and in other areas, it should be borne in mind, there were doctors whose earnings fell so far short of £2,000 that they were virtually in another League.

Purchase needed much the same capital sum as putting up your plate. The method was to buy a share in a practice to produce, say, £1,500 a year over a period usually of two to two and a half years. This meant an assured income from the start, but if the junior partner proved unsuccessful in attracting new patients, or even in keeping the old, his principal was likely to try to get rid of him. There was, also, the real problem of how the two would get on personally if they had not known each other previously. For these and other reasons, negotiations were normally conducted by solicitors, some of whom specialised in such work, and a partnership agreement was a long and complicated document, as, indeed, it still is.

It had to cover such imponderables as doctor-like qualities and behaviour, and the necessity of possessing and manifesting same, along with hard realities connected with reasons for dissolving the partnership – with the obligation on the partner who left it not to set up in practice within two miles – reasonable grounds for kicking out a partner and details of practice administration. It was well to be sure that the contract was explicit about death and retirement, otherwise a hopeful young man might find himself landed with a senior partner aged ninety, who showed up twice a week or so, and be powerless to do anything about the situation. The example is not imaginary.

The market in practices was conducted largely through advertisements in the medical journals and, to a much smaller extent, under the counter. Far from being illegal, or reprehensible, the latter method was a recognised way to what tended to be the better jobs. A doctor, or a firm of doctors, with a vacancy for a junior, passed on the information to his or their old teaching hospital, or the Dean of the Medical School, or a former chief. Since anybody doing so was likely to be confident that he had a good thing to offer, prices tended to be higher than the average. It was the bespoke end of the trade.

The medical journals teemed with advertisements from practices looking for juniors or assistants and from juniors looking for partnerships or assistantships, also from the many medical agencies which throve on these deals. The range was wide. A Grand Canyon of an abyss yawned between the London EC practice, 'average over £640, panel 500, rapidly increasing, visiting 3s. 6d. and 10s. 6d., no midwifery, small house, £95 a year inclusive, long lease. Could be run as lock-up. Premium one year'; and the Midlands partnership, 'middle and working-class practice, £6,200 a year, first-class hunting area, country town, panel over 3,000, capable, energetic man, cottage hospital, ample scope for good surgeon, half-share, two years purchase'.

A number of the advertisements mentioned the scope for surgery, or stipulated that 'major surgery' was essential, since the post involved succession to a vacancy on the staff of the local hospital. A number wanted qualifications in ophthalmology: it constituted 'nearly half the total income' of one Midlands practice. Such requirements are a reminder of the fact that, in 1933, outside London, full-time specialists were far less numerous than they are today and that many of the gaps were filled by GPs who had cultivated special interests. Anaesthesia was a notable case in point.

Among the advertisers seeking jobs, some seemed to be so well qualified that one cannot help wondering that they should have been on the labour market. Why, for instance, was the aspirant to an assistantship, with 'five years GP experience, including extracting teeth, VD, M.O., T.T., drive car, motor-cycle, M.B., B.Chir. conjoint, D.P.H.' free and available for interview, London or elsewhere, 'immediately'? In contrast to the details of practice finances, of hospital appointments and of general social amenities, there is what would strike the young doctors of today as a curious absence of information about the working conditions of the practices. Forty years on, the advertisement columns of the BMJ – in which not one medical agency appears, except the BMA's own personal services bureau, the agencies' place having been taken by executive councils advertising vacancies in their areas – are full of references to local health centres, X-ray and pathology facilities, the attachment to the practice of district nurses, health visitors and midwives, appointments systems, the existence of 'full ancillary staff' and, occasionally, 'five and a half day week, no nights'. Two new trends are shown by advertisements for doctors to do night work with the emergency services to which some GPs at times entrust their night calls, and advertisements for vacancies for the trainee GPs mentioned in the previous chapter.

It is not only in its practice advertisements that the BMJ of the early 1930s makes strange reading in the 1970s. There were five pages of advertisements for private hospitals and nursing homes, mental institutions, convalescent homes and homes for alcoholics. In a recent issue there were only three for nursing homes. All three were advertising forty years ago, but the space they took now was a great deal more modest. The only display advertisements for such private establishments were those for four abortion clinics. In 1933 the BMA apparently had no reserves about patent medicines – was the implication that they should be prescribed or was self-medication to be encouraged? At any rate, the journal of the Association carried advertisements for Feather's compound syrup of hypophosphate, and Valentine's meat juice, and iron jelloids, which would hardly be boosted in a medical journal today, though the Doctor recently noted that, sixty years on, the last mentioned were still being advertised on the risers of every stair of Slough station, as they had been in his childhood. Still more inconceivable at the present time would be the half-page advertisement carried in 1933 for cigarettes.

The advertisements for cars, new and used, make wistful reading. There was a 1931 16 h.p. Crossley for £155, and a 1929 Sunbeam, 'as new', for the same price. The 1932 Wolsey Hornet, a four-seater with a sunshine roof, was going for £185.

There were opportunities to acquire 'clothes of distinction for men of discriminating tastes, specially cut for each individual figure', at a cost 'no more than mass production'. Specimens cited were 'officer jacket and vest, black or grey, at four guineas, with trousers in solid fancy worsted at two guineas, ideal suit for professional or business men', overcoats for five guineas, a dress suit for ten and riding breeches for two.

The other side of the picture was indicated by an advertisement for a medical protection society, which had been established in 1892 'for the collection of bad debts without offence'. It was also apparent in details of the salaries which large, non-teaching hospitals were offering to junior staff. Typical was the £200 a year 'with full residential emoluments' for a casualty officer at a Midlands hospital of 500 beds. It was 'subject to any voluntary abatement from time to time in force', and the successful candidate would be required to refund to the council any outside fees received. At the time of writing, a Junior House Officer would get £1,914 in his first year, a Senior House Officer, at his maximum £2,850, with deductions for board and lodging for voluntary residents only.

The problem of raising capital to buy a partnership was solved for the Doctor by his mother's handing over to him the share of her estate which he would ultimately have inherited, and upon which, meantime, he paid interest to her. There were a few false starts before the business of obtaining a partnership was finally clinched. He had already received an offer from the old Eton practice, whose present principal had succeeded to the vacancy created by the death of the Doctor's father. It was a generous gesture and a promising opportunity, because there was still a little of his father's goodwill – that intangible which sent up the price of partnerships – on which to build. But, after consideration, both the Doctor and his fiancée decided that they did not want to return to the closed society of Eton, which was, if anything, more in-turned than that of a cathedral city. An advertisement for a practice in the Notting Hill district sounded promising, and the Doctor got as far as visiting its principal and his wife. The interview left him with a vague feeling that something was not quite right, but he was saved from having to make a difficult decision on such slender grounds, since the accountants' report was not satisfactory. Later, he heard that the departing practitioner had

59

been a morphine addict. The accountants also advised against an offer from the practitioner who attended the aunt and uncle with whom the Doctor had made his home as a student. They said there was too high a proportion of old ladies in the practice, so that the present gross yield of less than £3,000 a year was liable to fall, which seemed to be taking a poor view of the ability of a young man to build it up. That problem was settled by the principal's withdrawing his offer without giving any reason. He had an unmarried daughter. Could it have been that he had hoped to gain a son-in-law as well as a junior partner and that his hopes were dashed when he learned of the Doctor's impending marriage?

When, finally, the right opportunity turned up, it was through a variant of 'under the counter'. While she was on holiday in the South of France, the Doctor's step-cousin, daughter of the London uncle by his first marriage, met a practitioner from SW1. Two or three years previously his partner had died from appendicitis. Since then he had managed with an assistant. Now he was looking for a junior. The Doctor acted promptly on the tip-off. The first interview, in April 1933, went well enough to encourage him to go into the situation thoroughly. The accountants' report was satisfactory: the gross income of the practice was about £4,000 a year. Before the end of May he had signed an agreement for two and a half years' purchase of a one-third share of the practice at £1,500 a year, also his share of the fixtures and fittings of the communal surgery, which was reduced to £100 after he had submitted on inspection that they did not seem worth the asking price of £200. He was committed to living in that area of SW1, lying between the railway and the river, which he later came to think of as 'Pimlico proper' and to maintaining there an establishment, in keeping with his cloth, which would have a consulting-room on the ground floor. He undertook also not to practice within a mile of his senior if the partnership were dissolved.

The clause about a ground floor consulting-room added to the difficulties of house-hunting, which was already a little restricted by the fact that, to succeed in private practice, you had to have what was recognised as a decent address. Finally he took a twenty-one-year lease, with breaks every seven years, on a tall, narrow house in a Victorian square. It had the typical accommodation of basement with a large kitchen, servants' hall and various pantries and cellars; dining-room and two smaller rooms at street level; an L-shaped drawing-room, with two fire-places, occupying the whole of the first floor; the master bedroom above it and another bedroom, with a bathroom protruding behind as if stuck on as an afterthought, on a mezzanine floor; two more bedrooms on the third floor, and two servants' rooms at the top of the house. A ladder from the basement yard gave entry to a large garage opening on to the mews.

The rent was £150 a year, plus rates. Despite the encouragement of his lawyer, the Doctor recoiled from the suggestion that he should buy a sixty-year lease on the property for £1,800. He had a horror of going into the red to raise capital, and, indeed, at that period, it was usual to start married life in a rented house. Taking out a mortgage had not yet established itself in the habits of the professional classes. When he returned from service overseas, having given up his lease of the house on the outbreak of war, he found that the L-shaped drawing-room was now a flat, with sitting-room, bedroom, bathroom and kitchen, which was let for more than £150 a year. The two maids' rooms had been converted into a penthouse and sold for about £4,000.

In a July heatwave, when, on three successive days, the thermometer rose above 90°F, the Doctor and his wife moved into their first house. There was a certain amount of family furniture; with that as a basis, augmented by wedding presents, £150 spent in the second-hand, and kitchen and Household departments of Peter Jones saw the place quite well furnished, even if there were no curtains on the top windows to start with. In any case, the maids' rooms on the top floor were not occupied immediately, since the young couple thought they would be able to manage with a house-keeper only. It turned out that neither side was quite what the other had expected. The housekeeper decamped at the end of the week, taking part of the contents of the linen cupboard with her. She was replaced, a little later, by two girls, friends, found through a local domestic agency, who came as cook and housemaid. The Doctor bought a small black Wolseley Hornet six-cylinder, a respectable car for a young medical man and the first four-wheeled vehicle he had ever owned, and entered private practice in a mixed residential district of Central London under the wing of a highly esteemed family physician.

Dr Clarke-Foster, his senior partner, who was then in his early-to-middle fifties, had taken over the practice a couple of years before the First World War, succeeding to an earlier model of family doctor, an austere, top-hatted Victorian practitioner who had been driven round the practice in a dogcart. He himself wore a bowler with his unvarying black jacket and striped trousers; by 1933 almost the only top hat to be seen in the streets on other than ceremonial occasions was worn by a well-known GP who went round in a yellow Daimler with a chow sitting up beside him. Until the advent of his junior partner, Dr Clarke-Foster had done his rounds in a smart, chauffeur-driven Hillman. After receiving the purchase money he bought a Rolls and sent his chauffeur to take a course in its maintenance. Whatever might be thought of such behaviour today, neither Dr Clarke-Foster nor his colleague of the yellow Daimler was an exhibitionist. The latter, indeed, top hat and chow notwithstanding, was recognised to be an excellent GP, knowledgeable and sensible and hard-working. It was simply that, private practice being as competitive as any other liberal profession, having a distinctive trademark was considered to be an aid in attracting patients.

Even at the time the Doctor doubted very much if the Rolls boosted the takings of the partnership, but at least it boosted his partner's ego. There was no evidence that his own felt hat and brown suits, with coloured shirts and matching soft collars, actually did any damage to the practice, even if this was one of the faces of the future with which Dr Clarke-Foster could have dispensed.

The practice could not properly be described as a fashionable one because the area provided a true cross-section of the population. Hence, there was only a sprinkling of fashionable patients, some of whom had a high nuisance value. Dr Clarke-Foster was, however, a fashionable physician in that he never had any truck with 'panel practice', as it was familiarly called. Panel patients were those employed persons who, under Lloyd George's National Insurance Bill of 1911, paid a small weekly contribution which gave them the right to medical attendance and treatment and financial benefits during sickness. For those below a certain income level – originally the upper level was set at £160 a year, which, at that time, was the income tax level, and the maximum weekly contribution at fourpence – insurance was compulsory. Traditionally, panel practice was considered a little non-U by the better class of doctor, though, obviously, in country districts or small towns, the doctor saw all comers.

Instead of stooping to panel patients, Dr Clarke-Foster conducted the kind of double-barrelled practice which was common at the period. At the poorer end of the district he had a lock-up surgery with the brown lino, the board panelling half-way up the wall with spinach green paint above, the padded bench running round it and the school pendulum clock which were proper to what was indeed a cottage industry. Here there were two daily sessions from midday to 2 p.m. and from 6 to 8 p.m., where patients were seen without appointment and normally paid spot cash. The patients who belonged to what it is convenient to term 'the private patient class' were seen by appointment in the ground floor consulting-room at his house, where the dining-room served as a waiting-room. This, true, was a superior cottage, but it was the same kind of industry. Nor, where Dr Clarke-Foster was concerned, whatever may have obtained with some of his colleagues, was there any difference in the standard of care which he gave to the two nations. He was devoted to his patients almost to the point of obsession, to a point also, the Doctor later came to think, which was not always to their own advantage, since he tended to create dependence. He was uncompromisingly directive, whereas, from the beginning, the Doctor thought that treatment was a two-way business for which patients should accept their share of responsibility. Under Dr Clarke-Foster they had none: instead they received instructions which remained graven on the hearts of certain of them in perpetuity. Decades later the Doctor was still liable to come across patients who would eat only English mutton, bought at the Army & Navy Stores, because Dr Clarke-Foster had said that that was the thing to do.

It was not too easy to be the junior partner of such a man, since patients were reciprocally devoted, and might even go away rather than be fobbed off, as they would no doubt term it, with the new young man. But on this there was some comfort to be found in what had happened at the Doctor's first surgery. Besides being obsessional, his senior partner tended also to be secretive, and he had seen no reason to let the surgery patients know that the assistant who had been with him for three or four years was about to be succeeded by a junior partner. So when, at his first session, the Doctor opened the door of the consulting-room, half a dozen surprised faces looked at him from the waiting-room. The first patient came in, but when he opened the door to say: 'Next, please', the other five had vanished. They had come to see Dr X and wanted nothing to do with a stranger. At the time it had been a chastening experience, but, on reflection, the Doctor found some reassurance in the thought that, if the patients could have got so attached to the assistant in a matter of three or four years, he might hope to earn the same sort of regard before he was grey-headed.

Dr Clarke-Foster was a glutton for work. He did not countenance weekly half-days, though he had enough human frailty to ensure that the Saturday evening surgery was always done by his junior, and only after a certain amount of pressure would he agree to take duty on alternate Sundays. He taught the Doctor that a good GP should be always reliable and always available, and that he should keep his patients, not handing them on to specialists unless it was absolutely unavoidable. If you handed them on you were liable to lose them, and if you lost your patients you lost your income. To find patients, Dr Clarke-Foster was willing to go anywhere at any time to see anybody. Like many GPs at a time when better off patients were excluded from hospitals by inclination or the Lady Almoner, if not both, he did a fair amount of minor surgery, extracting deeply embedded foreign bodies, opening abscesses, dealing with sebaceous cysts and the like, as well as some gynaecological examinations under anaesthetic in his own consulting-room or surgery. He maintained also that a GP should do his own pathology.

The Doctor felt that the principle of holding on to your patients might sometimes work against their best interests. After Dr Clarke-Foster's summer holiday, during which his junior made twenty visits in one day, starting on the far side of Hampstead Hill and finishing in the evening at Ewell, (having at some point fitted in a surgery), he was quite sure that the distance-no-object idea was a bad one. As regards doing his own pathology; in theory it was quite practicable – it was what he had done in the evenings at St Thomas's –; but in practice it was different. The time taken in getting out equipment, cleaning it, hanging about until the process was completed, then clearing up and putting everything away, made the business uneconomic, and there was not enough work to give up a room to it. It made better sense to use the old-established Clinical Research Association, with premises near the Adelphi, whose charges were rather less than the two to five guineas normally asked by a private pathologist.

Much the same arguments applied to the minor surgery: the fee you could charge hardly justified the chore of getting out instruments and laying up a trolley. He was a little anxious, also, about the efficiency of sterilisation: needlessly, since in hospital one could have done no more than boil the instruments as they did in the surgery. It was before the days of central sterile supplies.

What the Doctor never had any doubt about was that his senior partner was a first class GP, however dotty some of his opinions and pronouncements might have been. When you gave your whole thought and attention to your patients, as he did, you could hardly fail to do good, assuming, as was certainly true in his case, that one was a competent practitioner. When, in the 1950s, the Doctor first heard Dr Michael Balint's dictum that the most important medicament that the doctor could prescribe was himself, his mind went back to Dr Clarke-Foster as a notable example of the process. At the same time he wondered mildly why Dr Balint should have thought it necessary to proclaim so self-evident a truth, which he himself seemed to have been born knowing. Certainly he was well aware of it by the time he went up to Cambridge. Could this have been due to the imprint of kind Dr Scott of Windsor on a wheezing little boy of three?

As in the majority of private practices of the time, the two partners did midwifery, which included ante-natal care. Ante-natal and child welfare clinics were already well established but it was not until after the Second World War that the middle classes began to patronise them. Between the wars, two vicious circles rotated about the clinics. It was claimed in some quarters that they had been set up because GPs were not providing proper ante-natal care. This was undeniably true, but, granting the usual proportion of practices which were generally sub-standard, the basic reason was economic. At a time when those who were not employed had no medical benefit, pregnant women of the less well-off classes did not go to the doctor, or, if they did, consulted him only at the last moment. But when local authority clinics were set up, GPs practising in the vicinity complained that their patients were being taken away from them. For that reason, there were narrow restrictions on the extent to which the clinics could prescribe for expectant mothers: virtually they were limited to vitamins and iron tablets. Similarly, child welfare clinics could provide only vitamins and help with milk.

The practice also did its own dispensing. Precisely, the junior partner did it. His duty it was to see that supplies of pills and paper and wax were kept up. There were eighteen bottles of basic mixtures to which the important ingredients were added as needed, sometimes because they did not keep well in suspension, sometimes because even so standard a remedy as cough mixture had to be adapted to the needs of the individual. As there was no dispenser, so there was no secretary or receptionist. Relatively few GPs employed either, at a time when the practice of medicine involved far less correspondence than at present, and when there would be, as a matter of course, a parlourmaid with streamers to show in private patients. Additionally, many of those domestics, even if their education had been elementary, were intelligent women who were perfectly capable of answering the telephone and recording messages. On the other hand, a chauffeur was the norm for a practitioner of any substance.

Records, as kept by Dr Clarke-Foster, referred only to private patients, and were pretty exiguous at that. Records for surgery patients he kept in his head. Neither habit made life easier for his junior when the principal was on holiday and he had to take on his cases. But if record-keeping tended to be primitive, book-keeping was complicated and laborious, the more so as there was a wide range of fees.

Surgery patients, whether they came to the doctor or he visited them at home, paid cash, the minimum being 3s. 0d. for consultation with medicine, 4s. 0d. with medicine and pills. There was an intermediate species of white-collar workers who were charged 5s. 0d. or even 6s. 0d. The rate for publicans was never below 10s. 0d. Nothing below 5s. 0d. was ever entered in the books: bills were reserved for the gentry. There was a special régime for single gentlewomen living in hotels, boarding houses or lodgings in Pimlico, who might be treated for 5s. 0d. but who handed over the money in an envelope, a reminder of an age when, in a decent house, the doctor's fee was put under his top hat in the hall. Normal gentry fees started at 7s. 6d. and had a ceiling of a guinea, the last for a home visit. Working it all out took a great deal of care and thought, especially as it was essential that each partner should know what the other was charging any individual patient, since they stood in for each other during the holidays. This was achieved by means of a code. The appropriate charge, in code, was entered against the name of every patient in the book in which each partner recorded the visits he had made, and was inscribed on the label of every bottle of medicine. The code was Watch for Me, W being one shilling, A being two shillings and so on. Sixpence was represented by V. The labels also carried the 'medicine code': for example, 8TNV v meant Stock mixture No 8, plus tincture of nux vomica five minimum dose. Treatments were seldom entered anywhere: the exceptions were a few patients, mostly the Doctor's, for whom there were cards.

The whole business of setting and collecting fees worried the Doctor a good deal. In hospital he had had the satisfaction of doing good – well, he hoped so – without being concerned about payment. Now he had to earn his living from his patients. Sending out accounts was not so bad, it was a respectably abstract proceeding; but he hated asking for cash on the spot and always felt apologetic about doing so. Even after he had decided how much, or sometimes how little, to charge, there was the further problem of deciding when, or if, one should go again; whether another visit would do the patient more good than the extra fire or food, not to say clothes or shoe repairs for some other member of the family, on which the 4s. 0d. would otherwise have been spent. He used to compromise by doing as much as he possibly could during his one visit, though he was never very sure that he had made a correct judgment about whether or not to return in any particular case.

But if collecting cash worried the Doctor, the book-keeping sessions with Dr Clarke-Foster drove him near distracted. They happened twice a year and involved not only himself, but his wife – a near-mutinous conscript – and Dr Clarke-Foster's wife and daughter, resigned ones. All five sat round a vast oak table in the ground floor front room, a sort of phantom dining-room – nobody ever ate there – which was consecrated to such jobs as totting up the coded totals in the day-book, transferring them to the ledger, adding the lot up and sending out the bills. It was the kind of house which had large areas of lincrusta, dark brown to waist level, dispirited cream above. The red plush curtains, with bobbles down the leading edge, would not draw because they were sham curtains, of half a width each, so when dusk fell the shutters were folded over, and they were dark brown, too. The walls were adorned with sepia reproductions of two Victorian master-pieces: *The Marriage Settlement* and *The Will*, both conversation pieces about dramatic revelations in lawyers' offices. One of the details which the Doctor was later to note to the credit of the National Health Service was that it brought the end of accounting sessions as well as of agonising over what he should charge patients. At the time, the fact that the account-ing sessions took place only bi-annually meant that the Doctor, being newly entered into practice, and so not yet having the security of a comfortable bank balance behind him, soon found that his money was not coming in quickly enough. With some effort he persuaded his partner that bills should be sent out quarterly. The idea of sending them out monthly was not to be thought of. Dr Clarke-Foster would have regarded that as chasing your money too avidly.

Building up his personal share of the practice proved to be slow going, largely, the Doctor believed, because his senior partner had insisted upon his living virtually on his own door-step in Pimlico. In that restricted area, a worker as tireless as Dr Clarke-Foster had already attracted to the practice all the possible patients. Had his junior been established a little further afield he was convinced that he could have done better. As it was, by 1935, his cheque payments totalled £921, rising to £1,061 in 1936 and £1,474 in 1937. In 1938 they dropped to £1,368 and in 1939 to £1,101 – Munich and the war took people's minds off their ailments, even if they did not take them out of London. It was thanks to a flu epidemic in the spring of 1940 that the total for that year was £1,310. Practice agreements normally entitled a junior to buy a further share in a practice when he could show that he was earning as much as the proportion he had already bought. The Doctor estimated that, had it not been for the war, it would have been about ten years before he could have bought more than his one-third share, which was about the average time taken to achieve equality with a senior partner. Today, when juniors no longer have to buy their way into a partnership, they normally expect parity, as of right, in three years or even less.

CHAPTER 5

PRE-WAR LONDON:
DOCTORS AND PATIENTS

When, as he was nearing retirement around 1970, the Doctor compared the London in which he was then working with the London in which he had started practice nearly forty years earlier, the changes which struck him above all were the absence of servants and the absence of nursing homes. Pre-war London had teemed with servants. When he himself had been established in practice for only four or five years, he and his wife had employed cook, housemaid, nanny to look after their two young children, and a daily char. Ten pounds a week had covered their wages and the housekeeping quite comfortably.

Servants came at the touch of a bell push to make up the fire, or draw the curtains, or show visitors out; though, even in the 1930s, the Doctor was struck when a friend whom he and his wife were visiting in Victoria Square rang for a maid to fetch her a handkerchief. Later, he was to remember the incident as the last occasion on which he had seen anybody in Europe expecting to be 'waited on hand and foot' in such a fashion. (India, where his war service was to take him, was, of course, another world. In Calcutta the sahib was virtually dressed by his bearer, and certainly dried after his bath.)

When a doctor was called to attend household servants, their employers paid, the standard fee being half that charged to themselves. Sometimes the living conditions of those servants were considerably worse than those of most surgery patients, however desirable the address of their employers. When he was called to see one of the lower servants at a large house in Eaton Square, owned by a peer who used it only during the Season, he found her in bed in a basement cubbyhole whose floor was littered with ashes from an ill-kept, boiler outside the door. At that stage of his career the Doctor was an impeccably true blue character, but, being still in some ways a rather innocent young man, it had never occured to him that people could treat their servants like that. It made him feel what he still calls 'a bit Bolshy', and he made no great effort to hide his feelings when he mounted from the basement to the first floor drawing-room to interview the peeress.

The nursing homes played a large part in the life of a GP at a time when he was what disgruntled NHS practitioners used to be fond of calling 'still a real doctor', and when private patients did not go into hospital wards. True, hospitals had private wings, but the majority of GPs favoured nursing homes because in them they remained in charge of their patients, and so in receipt of their fees, instead of having to hand over the former to a young hospital resident and relinquish the latter. With the exception of 'Sister Agnes's', now the King Edward VII Hospital for Officers, and the fairly recently opened London Clinic, none of the nursing homes had any resident medical staff. Most consultants paid one visit to their patients after they had operated; from then on the after-care was the responsibility of the GP. In the provinces his 'real doctoring' might quite possibly include major sugery. That seldom, if ever, happened in London, where consultants were thick on the ground, but the minor procedures carried out by Dr Clarke-Foster and his young partner made it worth their while to invest in an up-to-date portable anaesthetic machine. It weighed a good 50 lb, and, since few of the nursing homes had lifts, they had to hump it upstairs themselves. In much the same fashion, patients had to be carried upstairs after their operations, though not by their doctors. Most nursing homes had an odd job man who acted as porter on such occasions. That the Doctor should have given the anaesthetic to those of his patients who had major operations in nursing homes made quite good sense, since anaesthetics, with him, was something of a specialty, but it was normal practice that the anaesthetist should be the patient's GP, whether or not he had much experience.

Standards of luxury at the nursing homes varied with their fees, which ranged from a rock-bottom two to three guineas a week, for homes for the chronic sick, to the twenty or twenty-five guineas charged at Lady Carnarvon's in Mayfair, and the eighteen guineas or so which was the top rate at the Empire Nursing Home off Vincent Square. This, having been purpose-built just before the First World War, had a lift, X-ray apparatus on the premises and a decent operating theatre and anaesthetic room. All too often, at the others, the theatre was an ordinary small room with lino on the floor, which opened directly on to the landing, with neither anaesthetic room nor surgeon's dressing-room. The Doctor did not think operations should be performed in that kind of environment, and had a lurking feeling that nursing homes were not always the best places for the patients, but quite probably the patients themselves would not have agreed with him. They often elected to have their children's tonsils removed at home: the Doctor once anaesthetised a child on a kitchen table a stone's throw from the Victoria Hospital for Children. What he did enjoy about the nursing homes was the post-operative coffee sessions with the consultants. It was an era when conversation was still practised as an art, at least by the older generation, and the Doctor retains the memory of brilliant flights of oratory, studded with quotations from the classics, which, today would seem archaic. Apart from the entertainment, a young practitioner could often pick up a good deal of useful information.

It was outside the nursing homes, however, that his work became increasingly absorbing. For the first time he was discovering how people really lived. When you went into their homes you got to know them at a level which was impossible when both sides were encapsulated in a hospital ward or when you met socially. It was fascinating to discover the difference between the façade presented to the world and the true situation, whether personal or material. It could be even more fascinating to meet the odd individual who was, so to say, *durchcomponiert* – consistent all through.

As to living standards what impressed him more than anything about his practice area was the remarkable lack of plumbing in the houses he visited. The impression was confirmed when, at the time of the Blitz, air-raid wardens, surveying the local capacity for water storage, found that the number of baths was extraordinarily small. The few blocks of modern – modern, that is, for the period – working-class flats sometimes had a bath, but it was in the kitchen, covered by a hinged wooden lid which converted it into a table. The less modern were not simply bathless: neighbours often shared a sink and tap in a common scullery between two flats. The one feature which redeemed the flights of stone stairs and the generally prison-like architecture was that the flats had interior courtyards where children could play within the sight of their mothers and out of the danger of traffic. The surviving 'village streets' of two-storey houses, which provided a more human environment, had flush lavatories at the bottom of the little back gardens; the houses with basement, ground floor and one above normally had indoor sanitation but never bathrooms, unless, rarely, they had been added. The only plumbing was one sink in the basement and another on the first-floor landing.

In the old property, quite frequently, there were vermin. Mice, and even rats, and, of course, bugs, were commonplace. Bugs, the Doctor had been taught when reading for his Natural Science Tripos, were now rare in Britain 'except in dirty carriages on the Great Eastern Railway'. He remembered that lecture on a night when he was called out to a case of heart failure in a patient who was the much-respected managing clerk of a well-known firm of solicitors. It was before the era of diuretics: the only way to treat congestive heart failure was to relieve the distress with oxygen, which the Doctor was able to administer with the weighty anaesthetic machine. He was sitting at the patient's bedside, manipulating it, when he became aware of movement on the dressing-table. It was alive with bugs. What, the Doctor wondered, as he watched them playing hide-and-seek among the studboxes, would have been the reaction to that sight of the barristers, and even judges, who would quite naturally have sat beside the old man and chatted had they met in a bus at the end of the day? Bugs notwithstanding, he succeeded in getting his patient over that attack.

When he had been in practice for a couple of years, the Doctor began to take an active interest in the social aspects of a GP's work when he became a member of the committee of the Westminster Housing Association, which, like other housing associations of the period, had two parallel policies. On the one hand it informed public opinion of the obsolescence of the bulk of working-class housing, which, in Westminster, had been spotlighted by the flood disaster of 1928, when people had been drowned in their basements. On the other, by means of a housing trust, it provided alternative accommodation, either by building flats or by buying property which came on to the market and converting it to a tolerable standard, then letting it at a fair rent and continuing to manage it. The 'tolerable standard' of the 1930s was not luxurious. Each flat had its own cooking facilities and water supply, but two households might share one lavatory. At least it was indoors.

The Doctor was involved chiefly with the Propaganda and Inquirers' Sub-Committees. The first, in effect, was a pressure group made up of people who either, like himself, were in a position to know about bad housing situations, or who made it their business to find out, and who then helped the tenants to present their case to the local authority. *Picture Post*, which was then in its crusading prime, weighed in with a complete issue devoted to housing, with pictures calculated to shake the most complacent authority. There were traps for the unwary or the inexperienced in the work of the Inquirers' Sub-Committee. A number of cases came from the area just off Millbank, where the drownings of 1928 had taken place. The fact that the local authority had put a closing order on the basements did not always deter families from moving into them: it was, indeed, quite a sensible thing to do, since those in condemned property stood a better chance of being rehoused. But there were families who borrowed children to make their overcrowding worse, and sorting out the true from the false siblings was one of the jobs of the Inquirers' Sub-Committee.

Both professionally and socially the area was an interesting one in which to practise. Before the war, doctors who were in private practice in big cities often got a rather false picture of the pattern of disease in the community, because they were seldom if ever called by those sections of society in which epidemics usually started. Here Dr Clarke-Foster and his partner had an advantage, as they saw the poorer end of the practice at the surgery. Even so, they probably underestimated the number of people suffering from TB and other chronic disabling diseases, because the financial consequences were such that patients were obliged to stop going to a private practitioner, while those who were insured, when they ran out of their period of medical benefit, passed into the care of the 'parish doctor', a practitioner who worked under contract for the Poor Law authorities.

Up to now, the Doctor's notions of local authority medicine

had remained very much those that had been imparted at St Thomas's – it was mostly about drains and really not quite-quite. His spectrum was broadened when his old chief in the hospital's department of Obstetrics got him taken on as assistant for the ante-natal clinic which had been set up by the forward-looking MOH of the Borough of Heston and Isleworth – now Hounslow – Dr Nash. The clinics had become so popular that more than one doctor was needed. He went to help at a two-hour session two mornings a week, getting back in time for surgery. A little later, the Health Department added to its premises and he got an extra session on his own. Working with good local authority nurses, and sometimes with home midwives, who often came along with the patients who were booked with them, gave him a new slant on public health medicine. His eyes were opened still wider when Dr Nash talked about the way in which anti-diphtheria injections, which, at first, the MOH had done on his own, were lowering the death-rate from the disease, and when he learned that Dr Nash's concern about the diet of the poor during the Depression had found practical expression in starting a cookery advice centre which taught how to get the most from the least. His thoroughness went to the extent of having a film made showing how to bone a bloater, because fish was relatively cheap.

All that was some way from the socially higher end of the home practice, one of whose characteristics was the number of single women or widows it contained. Some lived alone in large houses, some with one, two or three daughters leading the unremunerative life of the Victorian age, with the Victorian combination of decorum and discomfort. Some concealed from the world a degree of penury which he was still too inexperienced to suspect until a home visit revealed the truth.

There were some memorable personalities among them. A sprightly, active octogenarian, far livelier than her daughter – the latter, rather exceptionally, had a job – was an ardent first-nighter and otherwise divided her interests between Patsy Hendren and Edward, Prince of Wales. She walked regularly to Lords to see the former play, and papered the walls of her house with framed pictures of the latter. There were two stepsisters sharing a one-room flat who, in winter, in order to save fuel, spent most of the day at the Army & Navy Stores. They sat in the members' rest-room, lunched off coffee and biscuits, spent the greater part of the afternoon strolling round the various departments, and finally ordered one fish ball, or one cold cutlet, on rare occasions one each, to be delivered, so that, by the time they were home again, their supper had already arrived. Not until the morning when one of the pair called him rather early, did the Doctor discover that the one-room flat had only one single bed, and that the taller of the two women slept on two chairs. He had been sent for because she had fallen down into the gap between them, her feet still up on one, her head and neck being pushed forward by the other, and was unable to move. When the Doctor lifted her he found that she was wearing the dark blue mackintosh in which he was accustomed to see her by day. Beneath it there was only a pair of combinations, with stockings rolled above the knee to keep them up. For the Army & Navy she added a hat.

In different circumstances were three sisters living in a well-furnished, amply staffed house which was the last place where the Doctor smelled the smell of country house breakfast that he associated with childhood summer holidays spent with an uncle in Northumberland. The constant ground bass was coffee brewing, and the methylated spirit under the sideboard hotplates: the variations depended on whether, under the cover, there were kidneys, or bacon, or kippers or kedgeree. But, apart from the gas globes in the hall and on the stairs, the only form of lighting in the house up to the Second World War came from oil lamps and candles. All three sisters had inherited the Roman fortitude of their father, a general. The eldest was taken ill suddenly: the Doctor spent most of the night at her bedside, and was there when she died, by the light of a single candle. He was not called to the house again until the second sister got broncho-pneumonia after standing for hours in the cold at the funeral of King George V. She had seen no reason to consult a doctor about a dropped foot, the result of an accident which had injured a nerve in her leg. Instead, she had settled the matter herself with a piece of black elastic, one end of which was attached to a garter, the other to the toe of her shoe, so keeping her foot in position while she walked. She, too, died by candle-light, of heart failure, when she seemed to be getting over the pneumonia.

The third sister, who read *The Times* from end to end daily, did relent to the extent of calling the Doctor when she fell down the basement stairs, not at the time of the fall but on the next day, when she had a swelling the size of a baby's head on one hip and wanted to know if she had done herself 'any damage'. The Doctor was able to reassure her that she had not: she had merely broken a blood vessel which had bled into the flesh. He did not see her again until a Sunday evening when she telephoned to tell him calmly that she had gone blind.

That morning she had gone to church as usual. During the afternoon her sight had become so bad, and her eyes so painful, that she had gone to bed. She had come downstairs for tea, though by this time she could scarcely see. Only because the pain in her eyes had become so acute that, to her horror, she was sick in the drawing-room, did she telephone him. She proved to be suffering from acute glaucoma, a condition marked by increasing pressure within the eyeball, and by the time the Doctor arrived it was already too late to save the sight of one eye. He was left divided between admiration for so much stoicism and regret that it should have had so unfortunate an outcome. When war broke out she continued to live alone with five servants, until a bomb which fell near by blew in all the windows. The Doctor found her in an air-raid shelter, surrounded by the five servants. Then, and then only, did she decide to leave London to live with relatives in the country, and exchange oil lamps for electric light.

At the opposite pole from that Spartan household was the household of an old lady living alone, ministered to by a large staff, whose well-being demanded a visit from Dr Clarke-Foster twice a day, six days a week, and often one on Sunday. She belonged, unquestionably, to the sector for whom the rate for a home visit was a guinea, but, on the principle of 'cheaper by the dozen', she was charged only fifteen shillings, which still added up to around £500 a year. The name of that old lady was to be written on the Doctor's heart. When, one month after he had joined the practice, Dr Clarke-Foster left for his annual holiday, he confided her with due solemnity, to the care of his junior. Before the end of the month, and out of a clear sky, she had a stroke and died. The Doctor was appalled, clean as he felt his hands to be. 'Honestly, I hadn't done a *thing*!' he was to say thirty years later, and the horror was still fresh in his wife's voice as she added: 'It was dreadful. We didn't know what to *do*.' There was also the point that, a few weeks earlier, the Doctor had paid two-and-a-half-years' purchase for one-third share of the practice, and there was £500 of his capital gone down the drain in a single whoosh! He wondered how often it would happen. Dr Clarke-Foster, on his return, was very nice about the business, being quick to reassure his partner that these things were liable to happen to anybody. All the same, it hadn't happened to him . . .

Later, an older, more experienced Doctor was to reflect occasionally on how such a situation could have arisen. The old lady was a Victorian relict; she was rich enough to have got into the habit of being spoilt and dictatorial; she was German and so, possibly, not totally secure and at home in England; she was lonely. And, at the beginning, probably Dr Clarke-Foster could not afford to say no to £500 a year. But the Doctor decided that it was always partly the fault of the GP when things got to such a pitch. By 'fault' he did not mean that a doctor was consciously chasing fees, but that, by taking imagined physical ailments too seriously, he might encourage them to be persistent. There needed to be a dash of nonchalance along with the reassurance which followed a proper examination.

Doctors in the London of that day did, of course, sometimes run after rich old ladies, or, more accurately, some doctors did. He himself never came across anything quite so flagrant as some of the examples described in the novels of A.J. Cronin, but there was an occasion when, at the direct request of the relatives of an old lady who was dying, the Doctor called into consultation a colleague who claimed to be a 'cancer cure specialist'. The situation was pretty bogus in itself, though the colleague was, of course, a qualified doctor, not a quack, but our Doctor was shocked to the point of nausea when, as they were leaving after the consultation, the 'cancer curist', looking about him, said: 'She's got a lot of lovely things. Why don't you get her to leave you some? You've still got a bit of time.' It was with mixed feelings that the Doctor later learned that the old lady had, in fact, left him a French travelling-clock.

Incidents of that kind were exceptional; mostly the work was honest enough, and, in some ways, more exacting than at present, since patients suffering from acute infections might need to be seen three times in one day. After-supper visits were more often made to such cases than in response to new calls. Infection which got out of hand often ended in hospital or nursing home, since it was apt to lead to some kind of abscess which had to be dealt with surgically.

Even something so banal, by contemporary standards, as recurrent attacks of tonsillitis could lead to an enlargement of the glands on either side of the neck which might become acutely inflamed and break down. It was difficult to distinguish these from the common enough tuberculous glands, which were usually the result of drinking infected milk. Precautions could be tragically ineffective. The Doctor had a woman patient whose state of chronic ill health was due to such a childhood infection. Her father, himself a doctor, had been so anxious to protect her from avoidable hazards that he had kept a cow to supply her with milk. Unhappily, in the period before TB testing, he did not know that it had bovine TB until the child, who had had the germs undiluted, became infected. After the war one ceased to see children with the ugly scar running from the angle of the jaw to the beginning of the collar-bone which was the usual legacy of operations to remove these glands.

Sometimes, too, there were crucial decisions to be made, as when the Doctor was called by a young man who turned out to be a Cambridge acquaintance. He had a temperature; he was feeling rotten. It did not seem dramatic, but the Doctor did not like his colour, and sent him into one of the local nursing homes. A little later its matron, a former Thomas's Sister, telephoned to say that he was getting worse and she was worried. The Doctor went round promptly, to find that the patient was heading for fulminating pneumonia. With the minimum of delay he was able to get hold of a pathologist, and they identified the organism as a streptococcus. Did one give an intra-venous injection of serum, which carried a serious risk of immediate anaphaleptic shock, quite possibly fatal, or did one stand by and watch the patient die anyway, as was very probable? The Doctor gave the injection. It worked in helping the patient to turn the corner of the pneumonia. The effects of the serum made themselves felt a fortnight later in the form of swollen joints, and urticaria, among other unpleasant symptoms. It meant day and night nursing for a month or two, and it was three months before the patient was back to normal, but his recovery was complete. There was a bonus, too. The patient married his night nurse; more than thirty years later they remained friends of the Doctor and his wife.

It was the last decision of such a kind which the Doctor was called upon to take. Not long afterwards he was called to a patient suffering from acute tonsillitis which was well on the way to becoming quinsy. Quinsy was nasty. It meant surgery to open the abscess, and as the modern technique of intubation under anaesthetic, which completely shuts off the back of the throat, was still very rare, it had to be opened without an anaesthetic because of the danger that an unconscious patient might inhale the pus into the windpipe. For the first time the Doctor prescribed some red tablets called Prontosil, which had just come on to the market. There was no need for surgery. Over the next forty-eight hours he saw the inflammation of the tonsils disappear as though by a miracle. So, in a flat opposite Olympia, the Doctor experienced the dawn of the new age of medicine. Shortly afterwards, still well before the war, came the sulphonamides, notably M and B 693, which, though it made those who had to take it feel pretty wretched, radically changed the picture of pneumonia.

Home visiting was made easier by the fact that there was less traffic than in today's London: the relative novelty of cars meant that if you parked yours outside a house in a working-class district you were sure to find at the end of your visit that pre-school age children were clambering all over it, leaving seemingly indelible finger-marks and, worse, boot scratches. It was a period when dark colours, on which finger-marks showed, were fashionable, and when a young professional man took pride in the appearance of his car. Car heaters had not yet made their appearance. Winter rounds called for a rug which clipped round one's waist, as well as a heavy overcoat, scarf and fur gloves. Out of consideration for his patients he added a small hand-warmer which burned petrol vapour on a continuously red-hot platinum coil. It saved the time that would have been wasted in asking for hot water, and you left it in your glove while you visited the patient. In any case there was no guarantee that hot water would be available in the small houses, any more than there was any certainty that electricity would be available in the large ones. Even after the war electricity was something you had to be sure about before a consultant had lugged an electrocardiograph machine upstairs.

After dark the streets were largely empty. Almost no cars were parked along the kerbs, partly because there was no scarcity of garages, partly because, if they were left outside, they had to have side-lights and one tail-light burning, however well the street was lit. It was such a strain on batteries if one was out on a midder case that, if the distance was not too great, it was better to walk, though it was not always advisable to be alone on foot carrying a large bag in certain areas. The Doctor was once cornered by two 'thugs' who wanted to see what was inside it, but they turned out to be plain-clothes police. The doctor's bag was no light matter when disposable plastic syringes had not yet appeared. Glass ones added materially to its weight, besides being hell to sterilise. Making up injections on the spot was hell, too: it was almost impossible to achieve the proper degree of asepsis when you were fiddling about boiling in a saucepan on the kitchen gas-ring the forceps to be used to pick up a tablet you had shaken out of a tube on to a piece of gauze. But that had been the method of making up most standard injections at St Thomas's, chiefly because of expense. Today's glass ampoules, which cost six or seven shillings for a box of a dozen, were prohibitively expensive for a voluntary hospital where every farthing that was spent had to be extracted from the public by appeals and the efforts of voluntary workers.

All in all, the Doctor was kept comfortably busy, as well as interested. Only, how did one define 'busyness' for a GP? It was said that, 1,000 patients would keep a doctor busy on private work. It was not made clear whether that meant that one was seeing 1,000 different people in the course of a year, or that 1,000 people regarded you as their doctor, which was a very different thing. Most private practitioners would have found it difficult to say how many patients they had, since at least half of these were 'floating', in the sense that one did not know if they would come back next time; and, if they moved house, they might not let the doctor know. It was fairly common to get a call from a known address and find new occupants. Panel doctors had a maximum of 4,000 patients, which, by present standards, would keep a man very busy indeed. The standards of the 1930s were lower, partly because patients expected less, partly because there really was less that could be done for them. Also, doctors varied in the time they felt they should devote to their practice. The Doctor knew a colleague, with 4,000 patients, who played golf every afternoon. In pre-war private practice consultations were usually sufficiently leisured and chatty to allow a doctor to pick up a great deal of relevant information about the general situation of his patients, but rather few doctors seemed to think it important to take any action about the mild mental illness, the depressions and the anxiety states which were so revealed. There was a tendency to slap people on the back and say: 'Come on, you're too young to have nerves!' Even when early signs of mental disturbance were appreciated – in the Doctor's recollection there was considerably less of it than he found after the war – there was not a great deal that could be done. There were no psychotrophic drugs, only the sedatives, bromides and barbiturates. Extract, or tincture, of valerian, was an adjunct of almost every sedative bottle, and disgusting it was – therefore almost the most important item in the mixture. Amphetamine had just been introduced, but nobody really understood how it acted. Shock treatment for depression, which was in its infancy, was first carried out by injecting cerebral stimulants which caused fits, but even after the discovery of producing the same result by passing an electric current through the patient's temples, the treatment remained rare until the 1940s.

The Doctor's own day involved starting work at 9 a.m., getting home for lunch, perhaps looking in for a quick cup of tea, doing a surgery from noon until 2 p.m. on three days a week and from 6 to 8 p.m. on the other three, and possibly having to go out after supper if there was anything important. When he had got going properly, epidemics apart, he was doing about twelve visits a day, having from none to four patients to see him at home on three days a week, and seeing an average of four or five patients daily at the surgery.

Even when one did 'midder' one had a reasonable amount of leisure, and it was during those years that the Doctor began to enjoy the pleasures of London which, for one reason or another, lack of money being a major one, he had rather

82

overlooked as a student. Apart from theatre and cinema – the 'talkies' were relatively new and there was a spate of films worth seeing – there were the Blum and de Basil Ballets, usually seen from the gods at Covent Garden, on which the young rowing hearty of ten or twelve years earlier became fairly hooked. Eating out was rather less common than it is today, partly because one had a cook, but when you did go out you could have a very good dinner at Castano's, in Greek Street, for a maximum of fifteen shillings for two, all in.

Free week-ends were mostly spent at his wife's mother's house at Slough. A sister was now living at home and the assorted friends who turned up for Sunday lunch ranged from far Left to farther Right. It did not shake established friendships, but the give and take contributed to the Doctor's social and political awareness, which, these days, was burgeoning. Until now he had always felt completely secure in his way of life and in the future of the country. There had been political changes, of course, like the Labour Government and going off the Gold Standard, but the country seemed able to digest them. The early posturing of Mussolini and Hitler did not seem very important, and you couldn't take the Italian invasion of Abyssinia terribly seriously. The German occupation of the Ruhr was different. It marked the first time in the Doctor's life that he had felt threatened. After that the feeling recurred when he heard Hitler's rumblings on the wireless.

Despite them, life went on much as before. The Doctor attended his first ARP lectures; the unemployment figures remained high; at every heavy snowful the local authority put up notices reading: 'Snow – Casual Labour', to tell the workless what they could do. They chipped at the frozen snow until 10 p.m. Munich came and went. The crisis, like all events which take the minds of the public off their small ills, upset the income of the practice. Like many another citizen, the Doctor experienced relief and guilt in about equal proportions after Munich, and signed on as an air-raid warden.

CHAPTER 6

WAR:
HOSTEL AND SHELTER

They were on holiday in the country when the war came. August had been hot; domestic help went with the rented house near Newbury; two fields away was a farm where you could buy a pint of cream for half-a-crown. There was nothing to disturb the sunny, idle peace except the unusual activity at the neighbouring RAF station. The coming and going of aircraft on exercise frightened the children – it was long before their passing overhead was to become as familiar as the sound of the milk-van. Their parents bought a few model aircraft to hang about the house, and once the two-and-a-half-year-old girl and the nearly five-year-old boy had their own miniatures to push around at will, they lost their fear of the real ones.

There was no wireless in the house and transistor sets were not yet on the market. As the situation grew worse they used to walk over to Downe House after supper – their own house was in the school grounds – to listen to the news bulletins with the Headmistress. When, on the last day but one of the holiday, they heard the broadcast of the ultimatum to Hitler which meant virtually certain war, the Doctor decided that it would be wiser if the family did not return to London. The next morning he drove North to Milton, where Dr Clarke-Foster had a house. The family spent the night there and the children stayed on over Saturday while the Doctor and his wife went up to the London house to pack the things which she and the children would need for a prolonged stay in the country.

They were on their way back to Milton on that famous Sunday morning, 3 September 1939, when Chamberlain's broadcast announced that Hitler had ignored the ultimatum and the country was at war. The chilly whooping of the sirens started when they were at the end of the Great West Road; almost before they had realised what was happening wardens appeared to say that there was an air raid on and they must take cover in a shelter near by. It was an unpleasant twenty minutes before the all clear sounded. ARP lectures had been explicit about the destructive power of bombs, and Hitler's reputation was such that dropping them within minutes of the declaration of war seemed in character.

On Monday morning the Doctor, alone, returned to London to shut up the house in the square, put the furniture in store and move in with Dr Clarke-Foster to share his grass-widower's existence. The servants had not come back: he had told them at the beginning of the holiday that if war broke out he would no longer be able to employ them.

London was suddenly blanketed by a darkness that was pierced here and there by illegal gleams where hastily improvised black-out curtains had proved ineffective. Street lights were totally quenched; railway and underground stations were hardly less dark; after lighting-up time, cars and buses crept along on sidelights only. After a few nights even these were reduced to a circle of opaque or white painted glass, one inch in diameter, in a black painted surround. Later, a single headlight was allowed, screened to reduce the intensity and cast the light down to about fifteen feet in front of the vehicle. There was little entertaining and, though cinemas and theatres continued, getting to them through the black-out seemed scarcely worth the trouble. After supper, shrouded behind heavy curtains, the Doctor played cribbage with his partner before going to bed early to read *War and Peace*. He was struck by the resemblance between Napoleon's movement towards the domination of Europe and Hitler's strategy. The book might have been a forecast.

The practice was dead: half the patients had moved out of London and the other half were too busy to be ill. There seemed no point in the Doctor's joining up, when there were orderly arrangements for calling him up when he was needed. He took his name off the wardens' list because it was obvious that, when the raids came, he would be needed in his own profession. He was, in fact, incorporated in the Emergency Medical Services as an anaesthetist and, had the occasion arisen, would have been attached to the hospital at Park Prewett, but this was theory only. Immediately, he wrote to the MOH of Westminster, offering his services. He was told that he was the first of the local doctors to have done so, and was detailed to give First Aid lectures to air-raid wardens at two guineas a time. He was not enrolled in any of the casualty clearing teams because his call-up would not be long delayed and the teams were staffed by doctors who would be staying in London.

The phoney war ended in May and June, 1940, with the German breakthrough, followed by Dunkirk and the fall of France. For the Doctor and his wife, even that tragedy was overshadowed by the agonising decision they had to take about the children. They had connections in the USA who offered hospitality for the duration, regardless of whether it would be possible to get money out of England for their support. Finally they accepted, and took the small boy and girl to Liverpool, where their last sight of them was waving from the windows of a bus which was taking them to embark in an unknown ship at an unknown dock: for security reasons no details were given. Numb with misery, their parents travelled back to London in a compartment full of people who had arrived at Liverpool in the last British vessel to get out of the South of France. It had been a collier so crammed with refugees that some were accommodated in a bunker, and the interminable journey, with the train stopping and starting because of air-raid warnings, was punctuated by the voice of one of the Englishwomen who, in those days, settled in large flocks on the Riviera, droning on about how black her bra had got. When they returned to London they found a flat in Chelsea, where at least they could be together, and moved in on to the sixth floor on the day that West London got its first daylight raid.

Work came with the Blitz, though not to the practice. That remained so sluggish that even when Dr Clarke-Foster, who was over sixty and was becoming increasingly edgy from the lack of sleep which was one of the side-effects of the raids, decided to give up and move out of London, the Doctor was able to manage it with time to spare. But the MOH was delighted to have available a practitioner who, because he was not a member of the casualty services, could be called on for a variety of jobs. One of them was helping with the arrangements for evacuating old people who lived alone and either could not or would not go down to the shelters when the air-raid sirens sounded. The Doctor went round to visit them and record the necessary particulars, accompanied by a woman sanitary inspector – as health officers were then called – who proved a delightful working companion. He never heard how the old people fared at the local authority hospitals in the provinces, to which they were taken by special trains. The problems which many of them presented or encountered gave a good deal of work to the newly founded National Old People's Welfare Committee.

The next job was more rewarding: in human terms, that is, since it, too, was unpaid. Westminster City Council had requisitioned empty houses, including that vacated by the Doctor, to provide shelter for families or individuals who were bombed out of their own homes. They settled a group of old people who, on the whole, did not fit in too well with younger families, in a large house in Eaton Square, with a woman warden in charge and the Doctor as Medical Officer. After one or two less fortunate attempts, the ideal warden was found in a queenly lady whose manners were as gracious as her carefully dressed and tinted hair was elegant. On both counts she was highly popular with her charges, and, in turn, was extremely nice to them. The Doctor visited every day to see that all was well, and gave prescriptions as needed, the council paying the chemist's bill.

It was his first experience of looking after the elderly as a group. He got on well both with the old ladies, who were mostly from the East End and so akin to those of Lambeth who had attended St Thomas's Outpatients', and with the small club of old men who were installed in the basement. One contrived a single bedroom by digging himself into the cupboard under the stairs, where he spread his blankets over piles of newspapers, which he collected diligently. Every morning he set out, with a small attaché case full of papers, ostensibly for the British Museum, to collect material for a book which he was reputed to be writing. Another old man paid court to one of the old ladies, proceeding from paying her pretty compliments to winning her heart by putting miniature bottles of brandy and liqueurs under her pillow. Suddenly he and she upped and went, eloping and vanishing into the hurly-burly of wartime London. The Doctor wished them much happiness wherever they were: such zest and optimism at their age deserved to be rewarded.

Running parallel with those assorted duties, the most considerable of the Doctor's jobs was that of MO to one of the air-raid shelters in his practice area. To a later generation one of the most remarkable features of wartime London must be the extraordinary troglodytic society which grew up in the communal shelters. Henry Moore's drawings of sleeping figures, each huddled within its cocoon of solitude as in the womb or the tomb, present only one of its aspects. From the outset the Doctor was interested in why people did or did not go into the shelters. Relatively speaking, safety was not the first consideration, or, if it was, it was illusory, since many of them did not offer much in the way of protection against anything more than flying glass. Most coal cellars beneath the pavement were designated as shelters, some even as public ones, and many people spent the night in them, or in their own basements, chiefly to escape the noise of bombs and gunfire. For the same reason the Doctor and his wife took camp beds down into the luggage room of their block of flats, because only there was it quiet enough to make sleep possible.

Many people who settled in big shelters, such as were established in Underground stations, did so for the sake of the moral support they got from being in company. That was a large factor with the population of the shelter of which the Doctor had medical charge; the shelter was no more than the basement of a large garage, still operating as such, which had been taken over as a sleeping area, a strictly accurate description for the conditions which existed at first. The floor was covered with ranks of people rolled up in blankets, who soon began to leave their bedding to mark their places. Families defended their territory as fiercely as robins. When, shortly after the opening of the shelter, sanitary buckets hidden by a canvas screen were provided, the family whose holding was thus encroached upon first refused to budge, then laid down their beds once more and slept with their heads against the screen, regardless of whether the buckets overflowed. After the first few weeks, when the place had become a little less crowded, the space was divided into dormitories by allegedly blast-proof walls, in each of which there was, here and there, an escape hatch 2 ft square of bricks and sand which could be knocked out. Flush lavatories were installed and, finally, three tiers of bunks round the walls. Social activities sprang up like mushrooms in the dark. From the beginning the WVS, now the WRVS, had been running a tea waggon in the shelter. As the months went by, one dormitory was used as a recreation room – there was even a stage at one end. When summer came the social committee organised outings by bus to Burnham Beeches.

In the early days – or nights – clergy and ministers visited the shelters as they thought fit. As the Blitz continued there were more regular arrangements for holding services and prayer meetings. By the time the Doctor was called up 'his' shelter had its padre as well as its MO.

Medically speaking, the Doctor found the prospect of being MO to the shelter daunting at first. There seemed so little that he could do, and nothing to do it with. But gradually things took shape. Somebody had left on the site a builder's hut on wheels; he appropriated this as a first aid post and held a surgery there each evening after the raids had started. During the day it was manned by a middle-aged woman air-raid warden, who became a kind of cleaner and caretaker. Sleeping tablets were less fashionable then than they have since become; what the Doctor doled out chiefly, by single doses, were palliatives like cough linctus and aspirin. As the weeks went by he got to know his new practice pretty well. Each evening he toured the shelter with a VAD, keeping an eye on the bedding and noting who slept where. People tended simply to disappear: when a bunk had not been occupied for a couple of weeks he got the City Council to take away the blankets, clean them and put them in store. As the shelter developed into something like a community centre he established a weekly clinic where he gave routine diphtheria injections.

The Doctor found a friend and ally in a City Council sanitary inspector who had an office in the Guild House, near the shelter. Mr French was cheerful and energetic and ingenious; the Doctor formed the habit of dropping into his office every evening to have a cup of tea and discuss projects and tactics, first padlocking to the railings the bicycle which he used at night in preference to his car. By good luck the two of them had already gone down below on the night that a landmine floated down on the Guild House and demolished it. It was the kind of bomb for which the shelter might have been designed. The inmates felt the blast and the escape hatches were blown out, but nobody was hurt. When, later, the Doctor surfaced, he found his bicycle intact among the devastation. He unpadlocked it and pedalled quietly home to Chelsea, through streets littered with rubble and broken glass. London during the Blitz was full of such bizarre contrasts. Once they had accepted Armageddon as the norm, life for many people took on an unexpected relish.

Apart from the absence of the children, the Doctor and his wife rather enjoyed living in their two roomed flat, where he had fitted up a small consulting-room in the hall. It was a pleasant change to have the place to themselves and not be dependent on servants. Outside, too, life was more relaxed and people were more friendly and informal. What it is customary to call 'standards' were abandoned; conventional women wore trousers and it was quite commonplace to speak to strangers. In general, the health of the people was remarkably good, although inevitably, there was a considerable increase in the incidence of nits and scabies and crab-lice. It had been feared that there might be epidemics if sewers were destroyed by bombing, and, in consequence, one local firm asked the Doctor to give typhoid and tetanus injections to its staff, but the fears were not realised. Through the worst of the raids London continued to be administered with remarkable efficiency.

Shuttling between the shelter, and the old people's home and his own surgery, where he attended daily between midday and 2 p.m., because it was no use expecting people to turn out in the evening, the Doctor was fascinated by the extraordinary remarks he heard from Londoners whose tongues seemed to be loosened and whose imaginations quickened in this world turned upside down. There was the elderly Jewish man who said seriously: 'You wouldn't catch me sleeping in a shelter if it wasn't for the air raids!' and the old lady who, giving a spirited account of a quarrel with her daughter-in-law, ended: 'And I said to her, Ada, I said, have you ever tried smelling your breath in an old glass?' There was the woman patient in his own practice who recalled a bomb story from the First World War. That bomb had fallen near a friend who was 'near her time.' 'She was so upset, all she could do was get indoors and have a good cry, and, believe it or not, Doctor, that baby was born with a bomb in the middle of its back, in the act of falling.'

The Doctor feared he had lost one of the more picturesque of his patients when, one morning, as he passed the end of the street where she lived, he found her house had disappeared. He had a special responsibility to Miss Claverton. She had made him promise to 'murder' her if she died, as he always thought of it; now it looked as if it might be difficult to open a vein as she had insisted. Miss Claverton, who earned her living by running a typewriting agency in the City, where she employed seven sisters as clerks, found fulfilment in other ways. She was a vegetarian, an anti-vivisectionist and a militant member of the RSPCA, apt to go into action with her umbrella against carters whom she considered to be ill-treating their horses. She would then mount the dray to harangue the crowd which gathered, and finally collapse with an attack of angina into the arms of the policeman who came to intervene. But Miss Claverton had survived. She had left the house because she was disturbed by particularly violent noise, and was a short distance away when she was knocked face downwards by the blast of the bomb which demolished it. Very sensibly she lay where she had fallen until she was helped up, when she went first to shelter then to stay with friends.

The Doctor's call-up papers came in mid-July 1941. He had had previous notice and had been offered a choice of Service. He had no very clear motives for opting for the RAF. It may have been partly because of a pleasant acquaintanceship with a retired squadron-leader in his block of flats, partly because he thought that, being the youngest of the three Services, it might be the most go-ahead. Call-up meant a further reduction in income. The Doctor tried to find somebody to take over his practice on a fifty-fifty basis while he was away, but an attempted arrangement with a woman colleague did not work out and he had to shut up shop. He relinquished the lease of the Chelsea flat and his wife went to live with relatives in Cambridge. The shelter community gave him a silver cigarette case (in 1941 doctors had not yet given up smoking), the VADs in Chelsea, and in the Abbey, to whom he had lectured, gave him a shaving mirror in a case. The old people at Eaton Square added to their farewells and blessings an autograph album in which each had written his or her name and a message of thanks and good wishes. H.M. Government gave him a £50 uniform grant which did not cover the cost of the items required. He took the train for Harrogate to learn to be an efficient RAF Medical Officer and left the shooting war behind him for the duration.

CHAPTER 7

SERVICE MEDICINE:
HOME AND ABROAD

Harrogate was like school, with four beds to a dorm, but on the whole more civilised. The medical intake came about twenty at a time for a fortnight's course on how to behave on a parade ground, which contained little that was new to those who had done their stint in the OTC, along with some elementary aviation medicine and an introduction to the forms and formalities of Service medicine. The lecturer stressed the point that Medical Officers should not hesitate to say what they felt about matters affecting health and efficiency. Later experience was to convince the Doctor that the RAF medical staff were a good deal better at opening their mouths wide on such subjects than were their colleagues in the older Services, who, at times, seemed resigned to the idea that nobody would take much notice if they did. It was one of the factors that strengthened his conviction that he had made the right choice of Service.

After Harrogate came a pastoral interlude at Credenhill, in the undulating, wooded country West of Hereford, where 7,000 electricians were in training. Work was instructive and congenial, if not exciting. The sick parade was mostly of trivial ailments; but there was a quota of mild psychiatric cases, men who had been so disturbed by the upheaval in their lives effected by the call-up that they needed sympathetic handling, supplemented by the phenobarbitone which, then, was the standard treatment for such conditions. A minor epidemic of food poisoning might have been planned as a picture book illustration of the dangers to be guarded against in mass cookery. The cooks came on duty at 5 a.m. and got going on the shepherd's pies which were to be eaten at midday. The pies were partly cooked, then left standing in a warm atmosphere before the final heating up. In those few hours the staphylococcal organisms which one of the cooks, who had a sore place on his hand, deposited in a couple of the pies had achieved quite a respectable growth.

The Doctor found quarters in the small house of the schoolmaster at a village five miles from the camp, and his wife came over from Cambridge. There were feather beds and an earth closet; the garden was full of runner beans and at the back there was a most intelligent pig who had learned to lift the latch of the gate and come and root among them. The only rumour of war was a single distant crump which started the old cock pheasant crowing in the wood behind the house, so it seemed the more improbable to meet an Indian Army unit stationed near by out for route marches with their mule-drawn artillery. The Doctor's wife, waiting at a bus stop, saw a village woman duck behind a hedge at the soldiers' approach. She didn't fancy her chance with men like that about she said when she emerged.

Autumn brought a plague of daddy-long-legs and the return of the schoolmaster. Briefly the Doctor moved back into the mess before being posted to Flying Training Command at South Cerney, near Cirencester, as PA to the Group SMO, which meant being the office stooge. He learned how a group was run, and, under the guidance of the sergeant in charge, how to handle a filing system. He had his first flight with an instructor in an uncomfortable Puss Moth, purely for recreation – he was not to be one of those envied RAF Medical Officers who achieved flying status. Once more he found married quarters, this time a sitting-room, bedroom and kitchen in the country house of one of the Cripps family. The Crippses were very kind, but it was a bitter winter and their house was mortally cold: the Doctor and his wife lived mostly in the kitchen, which had once been a pantry and where now an oil cooker thawed things out a little.

A three-day visit to Farnborough for the 'oxygen course', as the training in the physiology of high flying was known, was the one break in the uneventful daily routine. It was based on the very sound idea that doctors would be able to explain more convincingly to pilots the dangers of not using oxygen at 18,000 feet if they had personal experience of the effects of failing to do so. Three days of lectures and demonstrations ended with a session in the decompression chamber. The MOs entered it in groups of eight or so, all but one wearing oxygen masks. The one who had been instructed not to put his on was set to write his name and address over and over again. His companions watched him become less and less capable of doing so as the air was pumped out of the chamber to simulate a fairly rapid climb to 18,000 feet, until, finally, he slumped forward over the table, unconscious. The man next to him put on his mask for him; within seconds consciousness returned, within minutes he was back to normal. Each man did it in turn: it was the oddest party the Doctor had ever attended. The experience was not particularly disagreeable and there were no ill effects; the sensation was like undergoing an anaesthetic, though the recovery was not nearly so unpleasant. One man emptied his bladder, a common enough happening under an anaesthetic. It was a striking demonstration of the manner in which, above about 12,000–14,000 feet, without oxygen, one became progressively less efficient, and if a pilot lost control of his machine it was a toss-up whether he could regain it in time. Undoubtedly some crashes in high combat happened in that way, but more serious was the unrecognised loss of efficiency, which resulted in bad navigation and impaired alertness, with the resulting danger of being surprised by enemy aircraft.

Early in February the Doctor found his name on the list for overseas, and went to Halton for a fortnight's course in tropical medicine, which was good and comprehensive. His posting to India came through almost immediately it was over; he drew his tropical kit before going on embarkation leave. Officers' camp kit included a canvas bed on a stand, washstand and basin and canvas bucket. The Doctor disliked a good deal the revolver that went with the equipment. It was hardly possible to pretend that revolvers were purely ornamental, like swords. They were for killing people with, and he had always felt he should apologise if he even hurt anybody. He could only hope that training and the gang spirit would put him into the proper frame of mind if it ever came to the crunch. In fact, though, like all MOs, he underwent some preliminary training in its use, he neither wore it nor was expected to wear it except when travelling by train in India. It was statutory then, presumably so that one would have some personal prectection in the event of civilian riots, which, at that time, were a very real possibility. He was to remain doubtful about the principle of revolvers for MOs, which he felt to be a contravention of the Geneva Convention.

Back in Cambridge he arranged to sell his car, which had gone with him from camp to camp, and took train for Liverpool through an ironbound landscape with ditches full of ice. There was an hour to wait at Bletchley – memories of wartime Britain are studded with waits at Bletchley, many of them longer than an hour –, and a crated foxhound, who was clearly feeling as miserable as the Doctor himself, howled the whole time. A blizzard was raging when he arrived at the hutted camp on the Wirral Peninsula. There were days to wait with nothing to do except see the sights of bombed Liverpool before, on 14 March, they sailed for the Clyde, where they waited twenty-four hours for their convoy before sailing out again. It was not a bit like the Departure of a Troopship as it had been represented on the first gramophone record the Doctor had ever heard. That one had been going to the Boer War, and there were bands playing, and people cheering and singing and shouting last messages. But it was possible that the *Johann Van Olden Barnveld*, in which the Doctor sailed, was a more comfortable ship. She was a slap-up, 20,000-ton Netherlands liner, with a Dutch crew, Malay stewards, a lot of teak panelling and four square meals a day, meals such as her passengers had not seen since the beginning of the war. After trooping throughout the war, she was handed back to the Dutch, who sold her to the Greeks. The ship that had survived the landings in Italy and North Africa ended in disaster and shame when, turned into a cruising liner and re-named *Lakonia*, she caught fire north of Madeira on 22 December 1963, and was abandoned with the loss of 124 lives.

Officers had cabins with four or six berths, bathrooms with hot and cold sea water and unlimited drink. Other ranks inhabited a different world: sleeping in hammocks in the hold, with messdeck benches, drawing food in pannikins from a central point and queueing in the canteen for beer and cigarettes, both of which were rather scarce. In their leisure they lay about the decks playing housey-housey. Egalitarian ideas had not yet tainted the Forces in the spring of 1942. Some of the officers had even been issued with pamphlets on what to expect when they got to India, how much to pay one's bearer, how many polo ponies one could keep on one's pay, the chances of tiger-shooting and so on. Neither polo nor shooting tigers being among the Doctor's preferred forms of recreation, he looked about for the other components of a bridge four – he had scarcely played since he was a medical student – and settled down to what was to be his chief leisure occupation for the whole of his time overseas. It kept you out of mischief and stopped you spending money.

There were some Army on board, but the *Johann Van Olden* was an RAF ship, and, at the outset, the senior RAF Medical Officer assembled his staff and announced that they would run the medical side without help from the other Services. They established a rota for the sick parade and for looking after the hospital. Most of the work was TAB reactions and some odds and ends due to overcrowding. It all worked out very well until they got to Freetown, where a man developed acute appendicitis on Easter Monday – so, even in the South Atlantic, the Doctor noted with interest, abdominal emergencies always happened on bank holidays. There was an abundance of RAF doctors, there was an RAF anaesthetist in himself, but the RAF could not provide anybody for the cutting and tacking. They had to borrow a surgeon from the Army. Since there was no modern apparatus, the anaesthetic, perforce, was good, old-fashioned chloroform and ether. In the prevailing high temperature the stuff evaporated so rapidly that, when administering it, it was difficult to anaesthetise the patient without at the same time laying out the surgical team. The Doctor managed it by using a complete bath towel to cover the gamgee mask, in order to prevent the vapour from disappearing and to make sure that the patient got it. Not only was the operation successful, but the patient made a good recovery.

After Cape Town, where they had three days' shore leave and were royally fêted by the British section of the population, the convoy scattered for the various sections of the Far East theatre, other than Singapore, which had already fallen. The *Johann Van Olden* was for Bombay. With the troops now dressed in tropical kit of khaki shorts, shirt and topee of the same pattern as in the time of Lord Roberts, she sailed up the East Coast of Africa to Durban and then across the Indian Ocean, two officers short. One had fallen downstairs while very drunk and had the bad luck to crash his head on the newel post at the bottom, with fatal results. The second, who had gone missing because of entanglements with women in Cape Town, arrived in Bombay before them, having made the passage under arrest in the *Queen Mary*.

Bombay in May was seething and dirty; the only lasting impression the Doctor retained was of the harsh cawing of crows who never shut their beaks because their only way of losing heat, as humans do by sweating, was to pant with their beaks open. In the tented transit camp you had to remember to pull down your shorts before sitting in a wicker chair, because there was a bug in every joint, and even if you did remember you still got bitten. The only home thought in this abroad was the Army & Navy Stores, which reproduced faithfully the atmosphere of the mother house in Victoria Street. On the seemingly endless train journey to Delhi, across a semi-cultivated desert punctuated here and there with biblical wells, even two panes of glass, plus a fine-mesh wire screen and a blind or shutter, were not enough to keep out the dust. They arrived in the stifling dark, where everything you touched was hotter than you were yourself.

The Doctor was chosen to remain in Delhi as Medical Officer to HQ; his colleagues were dispersed to Ceylon, Central India or the area around Calcutta, which was threatened by the Japanese. He got the statutory Delhi belly over quickly, then settled to the charge of a new practice. The officers were quartered in decent, rapidly built huts; or they organised billets for themselves in civilian bungalows. Other ranks were on part of the racecourse, next to the horses, in cadjan huts, frame huts with plaited palm leaves threaded through the structure. These huts were reasonably cool but let in the dust, as the Doctor knew from experience, since his medical inspection room was similarly built. Soon, the Irwin Sports Stadium was opened for the troops, so the Doctor looked after that, too, besides doing an afternoon round of visits to families in bungalows, or officers sick in billets.

Two days a week he was up at 5 a.m. to watch training in parachute jumping, since it was obligatory for an MO to be present. There were two Handley Page First World War bombers, with holes cut in the floor, through which the trainees, mostly Indians, dropped to land, if all went well, on the area once used for the Delhi Durbar. It was a pleasant interlude during the coolest part of the day, and there were no serious accidents, only a few damaged limbs, though many of the Indians were extremely frightened. Ghurkas, when they were included in the exercise, were a different proposition. There was a legend that when, at the end of a routine introductory lecture, a group of them were told that they would jump from 500 feet on the following day, one raised a hand and asked if they might perhaps start at only 100 feet. When the instructor explained that they must be at least 500 feet up to enable the parachutes to open, the Ghurka said: 'Oh, we do have parachutes, do we?'

Medically, there was seldom a dull moment. In peacetime Delhi had been virtually free of malaria: war conditions brought it back. Coolies working on the building of huts for the troops swelled the formerly sparse population of the marshes on the edge of the Jumna river. The Irwin stadium was only a mile or so away as the mosquito flies, and they flew; though, fortunately, the infection that they carried was the benign tertian variety. The situation was complicated by the fact that control was in the hands of the civilian authorities in Delhi, who, for some time, maintained that the situation did not exist. When, at last, they acted, it was by burning down the rush villages by the river, so compelling the coolies to live on the building site, with the result that they brought a certain amount of cholera into the centre of Delhi. There was some typhoid at the Irwin stadium until investigation revealed that there was a manhole, leading to the main sewer from the lavatories, in the ground floor room that was used for preparing vegetables. It was a copybook instance of what could happen when buildings were put to uses for which they were never intended.

Leprosy was rare in the Services. The single case which came the Doctor's way provided, perhaps, the only occasion during his professional career when he put the interests of the individual in second place, though, in the event, the individual concerned was probably pleased rather than otherwise at the outcome. He spotted an Indian airman as a possible case and the diagnosis was confirmed. After a period in hospital the man was told he would be sent back to his unit, but the Doctor refused to accept him. He knew that the kind of leprosy from which the airman was suffering was supposed to be noncontagious, but he knew also that HQ, like all command HQs was particularly prone to receive visits from MPs and the kind of people who write to them, and he could not face the thought of the to-do which would have resulted if the presence of a leprosy sufferer became known. The airman was invalided out.

Dysentery and jaundice were endemic. The Doctor kept figures for the second, and found that, for some reason, he was never able to fathom, the incidence was higher among officers than among other ranks. Alcoholic intake had nothing to do with it, since, in Delhi, the standard of living was much the same for all. The one group which inevitably got jaundice were those having treatment for syphilis, who went to the hospital for weekly injections – the syringes were sterilised by boiling, which was not adequate to kill the hepatitis virus. At least there were no deaths from atrophy of the liver, but since there was no treatment other than lying in bed and waiting until one got better, a process which took at least one month, and sometimes two, the waste of man-hours was considerable. One probably got jaundice through poor hygiene, so it was a case for energetic preventive measures – true public health medicine. With the help of an extremely co-operative Provost-Marshal, the Navy, the Army, the RAF and the US Forces divided Delhi between them; MOs of the respective Services agreed on the standard of hygiene which must be observed and took over responsibility for overseeing the café kitchens in their respective sections.

The Doctor learned a lot about the underside of the catering trade during that period of preoccupation with boiling water and double sinks, drying racks rather than dirty cloths, and washing facilities for waiters which included soap, nail brush and the solution of permanganate of potash known through-out India as 'pinky pahny'. Inevitably bribes were offered: he hoped he was not being insufferable when he politely refused even a cigarette. If a place was persistently and consistently dirty the Provost Marshal put a Redcap outside to warn off Service customers. Unfortunately, one could not prevent people from booking rooms at any given hotel, and one of the principal hotels in Delhi, which had the reputation of offering the best cooking in the city, had also undoubtedly the dirtiest kitchen. It was the only place where the Doctor saw a rat in the kitchen, and also a swarm of cockroaches. When he picked up the lid of a disused icebox he dropped it in horror – its inner side was entirely covered with monster cockroaches.

The other half of the campaign consisted of lectures on how to comport oneself in a hot climate, which, in essence, meant avoiding the dangers of fly-borne infection by eating hot rather than cold food, washing fruit and preferably avoiding thin-skinned varieties. In fact, when places were clean, there were rather fewer flies than one saw at home, but there were acute danger spots at bazaars, where a man selling sweet-meats from a tray, with a fan to keep the flies off, had several squadrons on either side of it, which passed back and forth with each stroke, getting just time for a quick suck before the return stroke drove them away. On top of such obvious perils there were more unexpected ones. Europeans newly arrived in the Far East might be pardoned for believing that soda water was the safest possible beverage with the exception of whisky. Actually, every time the Doctor sent bottles of soda water to Brigade HQ for analysis it was reported to be undrinkable. There was a shortage of crown caps, and sweepers used to salvage them from rubbish heaps, rinse them in the river and sell them back to the bottling companies for re-use. Even in the officers' mess, infection which was pushed out of the door was liable to return by the window. An outbreak of dysentery among the officers was traced to the iced lime juice drinks which were nectar in that climate. The chief mess waiter gave the job of squeezing the limes to one of the sweepers, who squatted on the back verandah pouring juice into a jug. He had spent the earlier part of the morning cleaning out 'thunder boxes' (commodes), and there were, naturally, no washing facilities available for a person of such low caste.

The other serious risk was smallpox; the Doctor had two major epidemics to deal with. The first threatened to be a nasty situation, since it began with the accounts officer who had been paying everybody, but an all-out effort at re-vaccination damped down the attack. There were fewer cases than had been feared, and only one death. The second epidemic was more serious. There were forty cases among a European population of 10,000, and eight of them died. All who recovered had some evidence of a positive vaccination, if only in infancy; a single successful one obviously gave some protection for many years. Mass vaccination involved not only tracking down all the officers scattered about Delhi but also treating the Indian village with a population of at least 1,000, made up of mess staff and the personal servants of officers, with their wives and families, which had grown up behind the mess. There the Doctor went round with a team consisting of a medical orderly with the tray of equipment, the kitmagar who gave instructions to the villagers in their own language, and two or three beaters to round up the patients. The purdah women never came out of their seclusion; the kitmagar would stand before a hut and shout, and a timid bare arm would be thrust through the join in the curtains or, sometimes, between the two pieces of corrugated iron which served as the purdah screen. The Doctor would catch the wrist as it emerged, then scratch through the dab of lymph which the medical orderly put on the arm. You had to be ready to tighten your grip as the woman made the instinctive movement of withdrawing it as the needle pricked, otherwise she might have a scratch down the whole length of her arm.

The Services could present their own problems. 'We are not the kind of people who are likely to meet these smallpox cases', was the reply of the PA of a very senior officer indeed when the Doctor telephoned to say that he and his chief should be re-vaccinated. 'Indeed not', agreed the Doctor, and went on to improvise, with the dreadful fluency of a Victorian organist, on the theme of the very senior officer's dhobi carrying home his washing on one shoulder while on the other he carried his small son. If the child had smallpox, which was quite possible, the scabs – well, one would be enough, really – might drop off into the basket of washing. 'Just think about it', he concluded. The return call, asking that the vaccination might be done as soon as possible, came in ten minutes.

There was a break in the routine when the Doctor carried to excess his natural proclivity for learning by doing by contracting sand-fly fever, dysentery and jaundice in a straight row, getting up from one only to go down with the next. The first was soon over; the second put him in hospital for a week, with M and B; the jaundice sent him back there for over a month, and gave him a chance to learn a good deal about Indian hospitals in general. This one was run by an excellent consultant paediatrician, but, having only recently come out East, he had not yet realised that details of hygiene could not be taken for granted, as they were in London. There one would naturally assume that the lavatories were all right. Here the officers' ward was provided with two 'thunder boxes' not emptied often enough, full of ants and not adequately fly-proofed. The fly-proofing mattered because of the danger of enteritis, particularly as the flies had only to ferry across the courtyard to reach the kitchens. Nursing was in the hands of a few Queen Alexandra Sisters, supplemented by Indian ward orderlies who, because of the caste system, were limited in what they could do. They could not, for example, give bedpans: if a Queen Alexandra was not on hand, that duty fell to the sweeper. Caste apart, the efficiency of the orderlies was a rather variable quantity.

When the patient who had occupied the bed opposite the Doctor was moved into a single ward, the man who succeeded him got the treatment ordered for the original occupant. Their conditions were different, but both survived. It was a little difficult to decide whether the lesson to be drawn concerned the surprising amount of medication the human frame can stand or the irrelevance of a good deal of medication. The food was frightful, even allowing for the Doctor's jaundice, but at least it spent the minimum time in being transported and handled. At 6 p.m. a hideous squawking in the backyard would announce that chickens were being killed. At 7 p.m. one was presented with a grey mass called minced chicken and an almost indistinguishable grey mass called mashed potato.

The compensation was three months at Chakrata, which had been handed over to the RAF by the Army for use as a convalescent hill station. This was Kipling's India, as the Doctor had first met it in the books he had won as prizes at his prep. school. Chakrata was a flourishing small town which had been developed by Lord Roberts, with stone-built bungalows, though no water-borne sanitation. The country was marvellous, crowned by a view of Nanda Devi, plumed with snow. When the Doctor's legs had stopped feeling like spaghetti, he made an expedition to about 10,000 feet, from where one could see the mountain wall closing one end of the valley, with cloud or mist dropping over the ridge like water over a fall. There were monkeys and kites and eagles; on the hill paths one passed little trains of mules on which the hillmen brought their goods to market at Chakrata. One saw, too, the grimmer side of Kipling's India. The ages inscribed on the tombstones in the churchyard were mostly very young; death had come suddenly by disease, or violently in a riding accident – in this country, if your horse shied, you might go several thousand feet down the khudside.

Though he was theoretically convalescent, it was a working holiday for the Doctor. He was one of the three Medical Officers for the station and hospital, where, among more routine cases, one found the tragic ones of people who had got chronically sick with the bugs of India, for many of which there was, at that time, no very successful treatment. There was chronic alcoholism also, mostly among those who had spent all their working lives in India. One sufferer, an officer, was under close arrest, whether for some offence or as a necessary part of his treatment, with a sentry at the door to prevent anybody from taking in supplies of alcohol. He still got them, from the priest who was his only visitor.

It was in the hills, too, that the Doctor – who, though he was now in his later thirties, still remained remarkably innocent of the general naughtiness of the world; innocent, that is, in the sense that he found it difficult to relate his theoretic awareness of certain forms of behaviour to the living reality of people one knew – met for the first time the phenomenon of people 'going bad' when they left their normal surroundings and escaped into anonymity. What else could you call it when one Army officer managed to sell large parts of Burma to rich Indians who were naturally disappointed to find, when, shortly afterwards, Mountbatten captured the area, that they were not to enjoy complete sovereignty; or another appointed himself Army inspector of brothels in Calcutta, and made quite a fair supplementary income by accepting a modest bribe of fifty rupees per visit? Much willing more, he put up his prices to such a level that the brothel keeper complained, and he was nabbed. Perhaps going mad was a better term for the escapade of a fairly high-ranking officer whose engagement was announced in *The Times of India*. By chance somebody at GHQ who noticed the announcement noticed also that the officer was sending part of his pay to his wife and family at home, and he was ordered to go up to Simla and settle things with the lady. He did so, but, in the train on the way back, he was stricken with paralysis and brought to the Doctor, who referred him to the British Military Hospital. There, it was decided that the paralysis was hysterical: he made a swift and complete recovery and was sent home.

One incident at Chakrata, trivial enough in itself, typified for the Doctor the reason why, for the whole of his time in India, he was basically fairly unhappy, much as he enjoyed the work and sensitive as he was to the beauty of the country. One day he omitted to take his cigarette case – it was the one which had been a farewell present from his air-raid shelter community in London – with him when he went into the bathroom for a shower. When he came out, he found it had vanished from the table in the living-room of his bungalow. Later, he mentioned the loss casually to the CO of the hospital and, in no time at all, the local Anglo-Indian police were on the spot, questioning his bearer, on the assumption that he had taken the case, and frightening him badly. The Doctor, who was not normally given to anger, was annoyed about it equally, because his CO had acted without telling him and because it was taken for granted that his bearer was guilty of the theft. Anybody might have picked up the case which he had been so careless as to leave lying about. He refused to help the police with their inquiries, so, rather to their displeasure, they could not bring a charge. In the meantime his bearer, very sensibly, bolted. When the Doctor was about to start looking for another, a candidate presented himself. Munni was to prove a good and faithful servant who stayed with him until the end of his time in India. Had he volunteered for the job because his predecessor had not been prosecuted? The Doctor had an idea that it might have been so. But both the action of the CO and the attitude of the police were fair enough examples of the way many Britishers behaved towards the Indians. It was most emphatically not true of the Indian Civil Service, but it applied all too often to hearty British Service types, who, much of the time, were pretty rude to the Indians. They interpreted the rather submissive bearing of the latter as servility and, being presented with a metaphorical backside to kick, were apt, still metaphorically, to kick it quite hard. An Indian might not understand very well what an Englishman said. That was a signal for the Englishman to shout, so adding confusion and fear to the original incomprehension of the Indian.

The Doctor himself was bothered both professionally and socially by his ignorance of Indian manners and customs. It was hard to prescribe effectively for the families of the entitled Indian clerks whom he looked after when he knew little about their way of life, or what they ate. He was equally at sea about how to behave when he was with them. Should he, for example, have accepted or refused the drink offered by the nice family of an elderly Indian who had two sons in the RAF and two daughters who were not in purdah, though they wore saris rather than European dress? He had not, in fact, felt like a drink, but he was afraid to refuse in case the young RAF officer who proferred it might think he was being high hat. So he said thank you without having the sense to think what their religion was, to find that the family had no alcohol in the house, with the result that he was taken into the sitting-room and left for ten minutes while the young man went out to buy him a whisky, and the girls, in the kitchen, prepared sticky sweets which, in Europe, would not have been teamed with Scotch. After that the family sat round, neither eating nor drinking, and the Doctor, to this day, does not know whether he did right or wrong.

There were good points, of course, ranging from the interest of the work to the fascination of the insect life – he had a vivid memory of the first time he saw white ants swarming in thousands round the light, while, below, a great frog waited to fall upon them as they hit the bulb and dropped to the ground – but they were not enough to outweigh the unhappiness that hung over the country, or the heat of Delhi, which was so extreme that it impaired efficiency, or the despairing feeling that you were beating your head against a brick wall when you tried to get anything done. The war situation did not help, Singapore had recently fallen and Britain was at her zero. When he returned from the hills in the autumn of 1942 El Alamein had been fought and the Japanese were being held in East Bengal. The British Indians had hopes of seeing their homes again and the Indians began to believe that the British would not be beaten. The difference in tone at GHQ was perceptible. South East Asia Command was created in the summer of 1943 and Mountbatten flew out to take it over. Even in the improved atmosphere he soon decided that there was little hope of waging a dynamic campaign from Delhi, and decided to move HQ to the pleasanter climate of Kandy, twenty or so miles from Colombo, in the foothills of Ceylon.

When the RAF camp there was sufficiently developed, the doctor was detailed to go up with the first party to take it over, leaving a colleague at Delhi. The five-day train journey must have been one of the last manifestations of the British Raj, certainly as far as the RAF was concerned. Officers travelled in first- and second-class railway carriages, with a water tank in the roof at each end of every coach, never more than four sharing a shower and lavatory, and four good meals a day. Other ranks were in standard military coaches – with one shower and one lavatory for thirty airmen – living on road-rail rations of bully beef, bread, jam and tea made with hot water from the engine. When the second contingent came up from Delhi, the RAF accomplished its own quiet revolution. Rations and allowances were pooled and it was fair shares for all.

CHAPTER 8

LAST LAP:
INDIA, CEYLON, RUISLIP

Kandy was fun: it was like running your own estate. The Doctor was able to get the engineers to amend the plans for the lavatories and kitchens to suit his own requirements, and make garbage bins to his own specifications. The camp was in a coconut grove at Oonyawatta, a short journey outside Kandy. The kadjan huts on concrete bases were cool and airy, and the effect was like that of living on a balcony without any glass in the windows. There was no waterborne sanitation and some of the deep trench latrines were fly-infested. When the Doctor lifted the lid of the Air Commander-in-Chief's lavatory in the office quarters, clouds of blue bottles flew out, and anti-mosquito spray proved an ineffective weapon. There was one method that would work, but it was hideously risky. The Doctor poured down a gallon of petrol, covered the door, inside and out, with enormous warning notices, and prayed that no Air Vice Marshal would go in and thoughtlessly toss a cigarette into the hole. He did not.

As the camp grew, the five wells which had at first provided water became inadequate, and it was necessary to tap the Mohawala-Ganga river. Since it ran through a big village half a mile upstream it was not an ideal spot at which to take a supply, but it had to be done, and the engineers did it. They built a miniature waterworks, with sedimentation tank, filter bed and storage tanks, from which the water was pumped to distribution points. Chlorine was put into the storage tanks and a chemical which neutralised it into the distribution tanks. An airman was employed full time manipulating the cocks, and pumping. Tests showed the system to be satisfactory, but one evening, while he was having dinner in the mess, the Doctor was horrified to notice what appeared to be a water-boatman sculling happily about in the water jug on the table. If that could get through the filter, what else might not be passing? As he brooded on the dreadful possibilities, he kept absent-mindedly picking up and dropping into his untouched glass of water the insects which fell on to the table after flying against the light. Suddenly one came to life and turned into a water-boatman. The Doctor relaxed as he realised that evidently they were water beetles which occasionally took to the air.

When it was not the cause of so specific an anxiety, the insect life, indeed the whole of the natural life of Ceylon, was absorbing. The night-flying insects in particular were fascinating. When the airmen became aware of the Doctor's interest they began to bring him unusual specimens to have them identified and to learn more about them. Once it was an Atlas moth with enormous Perspex insets in its wings. He caged it in an inverted waste-paper-basket for a morning, in order to study it, and found it had laid eggs. The Doctor kept them and, when they hatched, found some vegetation which the caterpillars would eat, and kept a spray of it in a jar on his desk. Unfortunately the resident musk rat got the idea of eating them and only three or four survived to grow to the size of his thumb before he had to move on and leave them. Sometimes the airmen brought snakes. Once it was the remains of a cobra which had wriggled under the door of a latrine on a dispersed site and caught an airman with his pants down – literally. There were masses of lizards, notably a lively one which ran up and down coconut trees, and a huge one, about six feet long, which one day poked an inquiring head around the door of the MI room.

More welcome than anything was the improvement in the atmosphere. You got more work done and relationships with the local people were more relaxed. A nice old man who owned an orange grove near the camp was inconvenienced because his son had now to go round the edge of it to get to school every day. The Doctor obtained a pass which allowed the boy to go through the camp, and the father sent him, discreetly small gifts of freshly picked oranges in recognition. He could not help feeling that, in India, the present would have been more lavish and would have come before the request. When the Doctor left, the old man gave him a brass deer as a farewell present. It may have come from Birmingham, but he liked it and kept it.

Perhaps it was the generally easier climate which made possible an idyllic interlude when the Command Welfare Officer invited him on a trip to the outlying islands. The Doctor managed to find a locum to stand in for him, and they went by jeep to the South, where there was a Catalina flying boat station, then flew another 1,000 miles to Diego Garcia, touching at the Maldives on the way. Diego Garcia was straight out of Conrad, a coral reef surrounding a large lagoon, a jetty with a manager's house and a population making copra. Now it was a Catalina outpost, the manager's house was the officers' mess and the airmen lived in specially built huts. Fuelling was done by lines of airmen passing petrol cans along the jetty. There was no MO, just a medical orderly corporal known as the Doc. Once there had been an Army unit to defend the island against invasion, and a tented Indian Army hospital was sent there to serve it, but, military administration being what it sometimes is, the Army was withdrawn in the ship that brought the hospital. The hospital stayed but the RAF would not report sick to it, preferring its own Doc. During three months only one airman was a patient there.

The Doctor and the Command Welfare Officer revelled in a self-contained paradise where the only pests were landcrabs. They swam in the warm water of the lagoon and feasted on blind roast sucking pig – there were pigs on Diego Garcia, most of which, for some inexplicable reason, were born blind. After three days they flew on to the Seychelles, where the Welfare Officer, a Group Captain, wanted to investigate the prospects for retirement. When they arrived back in Ceylon he got into a monumental row for flying outside his command. For once the Doctor, who had gone merely for the ride, rejoiced at having no responsibility. Even if he had had, Diego Garcia would have been worth paying for.

In Ceylon, even more than in India, the Doctor had time to think pretty deeply about the changes in his profession which were going on at home. Details of clinical developments were few and imprecise in the Far East. There were rumours of a new wonder drug so scarce and precious that it was used only in hospital for battle casualties, but nobody seemed to know its name. As he was preparing to leave India for Ceylon, the Doctor heard that a supply of it had been managed for an

110

Army colleague who had become ill in Bengal, but he never learned the result of the treatment.

Information and, even more, opinion on the impending changes in the structure of medicine, on the other hand, were plentiful. Before he left England the Doctor had read in the *British Medical Journal* extracts from the Beveridge Report on social insurance and allied services. Now the journal was full of letters on 'socialised medicine', most of which were against it. After full consideration, the Doctor was certain that he was in favour, pre-eminently because personal experience in India and Ceylon had proved to him that not being paid for items of service made not the slightest difference to his relationship with his patients.

In India, towards the end of 1943, he had been running quite a busy practice among Service families quartered in Delhi, whom he visited in the afternoons after he had dealt with sick parades and paper work. He had enjoyed it. Time did not press unduly, so it could be a fairly relaxed round, and there were always quite a number of children. It was there that the Doctor first tried the technique of drawing for them. He thought of it when palpating the abdomen of an airman, on which was tattooed a bathing beauty who wriggled under his fingers and assumed interesting shapes and positions as he pushed. He was amused and adapted the idea by doing moving drawings on the hands of his small patients. You drew a face on the back of the hand, placing it so that the line of the mouth came along the groove in the bracelet of fat which encircles a young child's wrist. When the wrist was extended the mouth opened, when it was flexed it shut, and you could arrange a little story to accompany the actions. That kind of game was entertainment after you had won a child's confidence.

Later, back in London, the Doctor was to find that drawing could be used as an aid in gaining the friendship of children. A quick portrait, readily identifiable by her spotted dress and the bow in her hair, worked very well with an intelligent little girl of four, who was deaf and dumb. It proved even more valuable with acutely shy children whose reaction to a doctor was to hide under the bedclothes and turn their faces to the wall. The thing not to do on such occasions was to use force or allow the mother to use it. The result was inevitably a battle and tears, which began again on the next visit. Examinations in those conditions, if not quite useless, were greatly reduced in value. The Doctor preferred to leave the examination until the next day and, instead, to sit beside the child's bed and, while taking from the mother a history which usually made it possible to start treatment, do a rapid sketch on his prescription pad of the child humped up under the blankets or even peering out of a cupboard. He would comment as he sketched: the child, almost invariably, would listen. 'When I come again tomorrow we'll do another one and you can tell me what you'd like', the Doctor would say, as he tore off the slip and left it on the bed. The next day the child was usually quite pleased to see him. The procedure even had some diagnostic value, since a child who was really ill would take no notice, while if it was suffering from one of the commonplace ailments of childhood, it would always show interest.

Practising in that fashion in India, visiting and treating patients who paid him nothing, providing medicines usually from medical stores – which were better stocked than the local chemists – the Doctor realised that he was already working in a health service, and as a paid official at that. Though he hoped that the British health service, when it was established, would choose to pay doctors by capitation fees (an annual payment for each patient on a doctor's list), rather than by item of service or by giving them an annual salary, he could find nothing in his present conditions of service that affected either the quality of his work or his attitude towards his patients.

He left Kandy in December 1944, when the position of being MO to HQ was up-graded to Squadron-Leader, and he was told that a more senior man must take it. The MBE which was a consolation prize – in later life he was to tell friends he got it 'for being a sort of upper-class lavatory man' – caught him up in January at Vavuniya, the station in the North of Ceylon where he had been posted. It was the first time he had been on an operational station, and as they were already moving out he had a peaceful three months in interesting country before his turn came to be repatriated after three years overseas. The return journey, which started on a low-loading lorry trundling along the jungle road towards Kandy

112

continued by train through Colombo and Madras to Bombay, where there was a fortnight to wait in a bungalow for transit officers, for his passage home. Bombay was boring unless you could afford to spend money, which the Doctor could not. The voyage back, by Suez, which took three weeks against the three months out, was equally dull until they were in the Irish Sea, when there was talk of submarines and somebody dropped a lot of depth charges. They were the first explosions set off in anger which he had heard since he left the Blitz in 1941.

Looking back on his time in India, the Doctor counted it a success professionally and financially, even if, personally, he had seldom been really happy. Professionally he had found Service medicine thoroughly satisfying. The only tedious job he had had was when, briefly, he had been full-time examiner of large numbers of Indians who were to be trained as pilots. It had been like doing an endless sequence of life insurance examinations and he never wanted to do anything of the kind again. He had enjoyed his first experience of having a mixture of clinical and non-clinical work, and had found great interest in considering the broad needs of the unit as a whole, whether the problem was one of hygiene – why was it that chasing cooks for cleanliness always sent the food standard down? – or of getting men back to jobs in the right way. He had no difficulty over relationships with his Service patients: their confidence and respect increased in proportion to the interest the MO showed in them. Even administrative paper work could be rewarding. Disgruntled wartime Service doctors, he had noticed, were almost invariably those who could see no further than opportunities for surgery or more advanced medicine, which were not possible in the usual conditions of station sick quarters.

Financially India had been good because the pay was half as much again as it had been in Britain. Since the Doctor had not indulged in any illicit money-making activities he was not returning as a nabob, but by living as cheaply as possible, forgoing expensive leaves and devoting his leisure to bridge, he had been able to save about £700, which was to prove invaluable when, in the following year, he was re-establishing himself in practice.

Immediately, there was a posting to Records, Ruislip, and

the problems common to many Servicemen who had spent years abroad, those of finding his bearings, in an England which had changed greatly in three years, and reintegrating himself into a family in which, inevitably, he was temporarily the odd man out. The children had returned from the USA in the summer of 1944. Now they were settled at Cambridge with their mother, well on their way in the process of re-conversion from a small American boy and girl to a small English boy and girl. Their father had not seen them for five-and-three-quarter years and they did not know him. It made the Doctor wonder whether anybody should ever be any kind of refugee if it entailed separation, or whether it was always better for a family to face its situation together.

Outside, the greatest difference was the loss of common ground with friends and acquaintances: one was in the position of a boy who comes back to school after term has started.

The relaxing of class barriers and the reduction of class differences had begun before the Doctor went overseas: in his absence they had accelerated.

The Ruislip job was less than exhilarating, though it provided medical interest from time to time when people came back from abroad suffering from tropical diseases. There were some discoveries to be made if you had been long out of England, besides the rediscovery of cherries, for which, when June came, the Doctor found he had an insatiable passion. Ruislip was near enough to Northolt to enable one to watch the flights coming in and out: for the first time he saw jet aircraft. They had never come to India and he was fascinated to see how they circled to land, travelling twice as fast as propeller aircraft. The wonder drug was in use and, at last, it had a name – penicillin.

Fairly soon after his arrival the Doctor became involved in a one-man crusade against Group HQ for a cause which belonged to public health medicine as it had been understood at St Thomas's – 'all about drains'. At an outlying depot for vehicles being prepared for the tropics, which was surrounded by bungalows and small houses, there was no water-borne sanitation for the detachment of men who guarded it. Every couple of days a night-soil cart went up to empty buckets, then drove through the streets of Ruislip to tip its reeking load into a manhole. The Doctor thought it most unsatisfactory: there

114

was too much handling; the risk of infection was increased by the fact that the cart was a rickety, leaky vehicle; and, since men at the depot were back from overseas service, the bacteria involved were likely to be exotic. He reported the matter to the Group HQ but though the correspondence file swelled, there was no practical result. With the war obviously coming to an end, Group did not think it worth while to provide water-borne sanitation on outlying sites. The Doctor thought back to the lectures he and his fellow MOs had heard when they entered the RAF. They had been taught always to co-operate in every way with the civilian health authorities. He reported the matter to the MOH of Ruislip, who thoroughly agreed that the situation must not be allowed to continue, and wrote to Group HQ to that effect. The latter were very angry indeed, but could say nothing to the Doctor, who was acting impeccably by the book. So the depot got its water-borne sanitation.

For the rest, they were quartered in small bungalows whose walls, one brick thick, were to feel like papier mâché as the winter tightened its grip. There was little to do in the evenings, and the Doctor, who was what people call 'good with his hands', took to leather work for recreation, and made gloves and a school satchel for his small daughter. The classes were run by the Education Officer, an amusing Welsh schoolmaster, whom the Doctor took home to Cambridge for a week-end because he wanted to see the village colleges in that county. It might seem as though, somewhere along the line passing through municipal midwives, by way of local health officers to elderly Sinhalese gentlemen who owned orange groves, the young man who made friends only with 'people like us' had sunk without trace. The Doctor himself would have claimed that he had always been able to make friends rather easily with anybody with whom he had some community of interest; it was simply that, when he was very young, northern grammar school boys at Kings and African students at St Thomas's had both seemed so unfamiliar that he had felt there was little likelihood that he would have had anything in common with them.

There was one break in the rather humdrum routine, when the Doctor was sent off to install medical arrangements at the camp at Great Missenden where the captured German Air HQ, which had been flown over to this country, was being held under heavy guard for interrogation by MI5. He went over in a van with a medical corporal, and found that the first and most urgent duty was to drive to the depot to get a load of sanitary towels for the women members of the German HQ staff, which nobody had thought of. Then the Doctor, still a Flight-Lieutenant, summoned the three highest ranking MOs in the German Air Force, all of whom were generals, to a conference to agree on arrangements for looking after the German personnel and ensuring that they had the needful medical supplies. They got on very well once both sides had established whether they were talking about typhoid or typhus. The Doctor was struck by the superiority of the German medical equipment. All treatments were in tablet form, in contrast with the rather antiquated British pharmacopoeia, in which the national addiction to bottles meant that, even in war conditions, one carried supplies of heavy liquid things, like cough mixture and indigestion mixture. It took three days to complete the job. When the Doctor went back to Ruislip he left the medical corporal in charge. By chance, not by anybody's design, he happened to be Jewish.

The Doctor came out of the RAF in January 1946, equipped with demob. civvies – being a tall man, he had the devil's own job in getting anything to fit even approximately at the depot near London – plus quite a lot of useful knowledge about tropical diseases, human behaviour, medical admin. and how to get what you wanted through the proper channels.

What now?

CHAPTER 9

STARTING AGAIN:
THE SHADOW OF THE NHS

For the Doctor, as for many of his contemporaries, returning to the civilian world was a rather bleak business. Professionally speaking he felt more naked than when he was born, since, for the first time in his working life, he was on his own, without the parental cover of hospital, or senior partner, or Service organisation. He knew that he wanted to go on being a GP, but he was not sure of the best way to set about it. He did not know if he would be able to build up a new practice in London before the £700 which he had saved while he was in India ran out. He had nowhere to live in London, and nowhere to practice from. He had given up the lease of his house in the square at the beginning of the war, and the surgery which he had shared with Dr Clarke-Foster was now a bread shop. There were some assets. His brother gave him a car, a plum-coloured Austin which had spent the war in a barn in Wiltshire. It was a blessing for, price apart, cars were hard to come by in 1946. He had furniture and equipment in store. Best of all, he had a list of patients, to whom he had written late in 1941, when the locum whom he had hoped would look after his practice had failed him.

While he considered what to do, he went back to St Thomas's to brush up his medicine. Those early weeks made three lasting impressions. The first was of how permanently hungry he felt when living on civilian rations, supplemented by what he could get at the hospital. The second was the introduction of pethidine, as an alternative to and improvement on morphine. It was, indeed, an improvement, but the claim that, unlike morphine, it was not addictive, was not borne out. The third was the cruelly Victorian attitude of one physician towards his patients. This was so intolerable to the Doctor that he avoided his out-patient clinics. Looking back, he decided that this particular man had always been the same; it

117

was just that, in a rapidly changing world, he was more obvious because he stood out like a dead tree. In his young days, too, the Doctor had tended to be impressed by Latin tags and apt quotations. At forty odd he merely noted that some consultants were so busy being clever that they omitted to show any human feeling towards their patients.

When his recycling was over he followed up some advertisements for partnerships in London. In all of them down payments were unavoidable, and the resultant terms of service quite unacceptable. For lack of any alternative, he decided to start up alone, to see whether he could pull together any remaining shreds of his old practice, and began the depressing search for surgery premises in an area of London which had had its full share of bomb damage. One small surgery was empty, but the doctor who owned it was unwilling to let, either because he wanted to keep out competitors or because he genuinely intended to return to it himself. Hoping for some useful information or advice, the Doctor called on the secretary of the local branch of the British Medical Association, whom he knew by sight but had never met. Dr Porter had more than counsel to offer. Above his own ground floor premises there was a vacant surgery and waiting-room, once used by his pre-war partner who, after demobilisation, had decided to do medical work of a different kind. It could be his colleague's if he cared to rent it. The Doctor jumped at the offer, unconventional as it was. It was not usual for a single-handed GP to be upstairs with a competitor on the ground floor, where he would have every opportunity of intercepting most of the new patients, but he did not feel that Dr Porter would behave like that.

Post-war London was already beginning to look a little brighter, and there were other indications that it was not quite the desert which it had seemed at first. Two of the Doctor's old patients had written to him at intervals throughout the war. Now one of them provided him with a bed-sitting room which, by chance, was very near where he and his wife had stayed when he took his first steps in practice with Dr Clarke-Foster. The other was to become his first post-war patient. The Doctor found a garage at ten shillings a week. There was no night access, but it was still worth it because, at that time, if you left your car in the street overnight it would almost certainly be swiped; also, since the lights must be left on, the battery would be flat every morning. He took his surgery furniture out of store and sat down in his bed-sit to write to all the old patients on his list. He would be lucky if as many as half were still living at the same addresses; but if the houses were still standing, and inhabited, the cards might act as a legitimate advertisement. Those early weeks were studded with long night marches along the empty Cromwell Road, against what seemed to be a constant East wind, carrying his bag. He could not afford to miss a single call, and, after nightfall, his garaged car was inaccessible.

That stage, happily, was brief. Before long he found not a house, but a six-roomed flat in a square very like that in which he had previously lived. It had central heating, a lift and no strings attached to the lease. He was not even required to pay the first quarter's rent in advance, but, even so, £300 a year inclusive seemed a lot of money when one compared it with the £150 a year, plus £50 for rates, which he had paid for his first house, or with his £700 capital, which was already eroded.

The first six months put an end to that kind of worry. That summer the Doctor did not take a holiday, and did two locums, one for Dr Porter, the second for another colleague, besides carrying on his own practice, where he conducted two surgery sessions a day. Also, he resumed his old job as anaesthetist at Tite Street, where the £400 a year which he was paid for three sessions a week, though welcome, was less valuable than the benefit of working with others. While aware that many individuals were able to maintain high standards while working in isolation, the Doctor himself found team work a great help in doing so.

A patient whom he looked after in one locum was a retired doctor with a very bad heart. He was the last sufferer the Doctor ever attended who got relief from using a 'heart table'. That now outmoded piece of furniture was a kind of bed table on which cardiac patients who had to spend their nights propped up in bed leaned their arms. By coincidence, he turned out to be the practitioner who had attended the Doctor's mother at his birth.

Patients, now, were coming in quickly. With some vague idea that it might ease the transition into the new health

119

service which was on the horizon – actually it did not affect the issue – the Doctor decided that, from the first, he would take panel patients. In the event they did not come in any great number, but their families, who were still not insured, did. His link with Tite Street brought him a large number of child patients, who continued the educative process which had started for him when he was a young resident at the Victoria Hospital.

The Doctor had always talked to child patients, even when they were as young as three months, practising with patter when giving an anaesthetic. Infants, he found, enjoyed speech even before they understood it, especially if they had talkative mothers. Now he greeted his young patients as equals on arrival, then gave them a short time to settle down and decide that nothing very awful was likely to happen to them, while he had a friendly chat with their mothers. There were toys in one drawer of his desk: a tractor, an ambulance, a ship in a snowstorm, something that made a noise when you rolled it. He showed the child the drawer and let it choose what it wanted, making it a routine that, at the end of the consultation, the child put the toys back. At the next visit it was interesting to notice which children went confidently to the right drawer.

Besides talking, he listened to the children. It was not always easy, for mothers tended to answer for their children, and also tended to dress and undress them long after it was necessary, sometimes, indeed, when they were young teenagers. It happened to boys rather than to girls and was sometimes extended even to husbands, when it was always accepted quite passively. He was struck also by how often mothers would say of a child: 'I didn't like to bother you, Doctor, because I thought she – or he – was only playing up.' In the Doctor's experience children did not 'play up'. Equally with adults they might be sick or have pains in the tummy from apprehension and fear, but a psychosomatic illness was not 'playing up'. When they were difficult and bad-tempered, it was usually owing to fear, which had to be allayed before you could gain their confidence. Later he was to realise how much his rather conscious development of a technique for his relations with his child patients had helped him, less consciously, to develop a technique for adults. They, too, metaphorically ran away or hid under the bedclothes when they were frightened, and you had to make a delicate approach which was usually a more complicated business than drawing on a prescription pad or keeping toy tractors in the drawer of your desk.

Altogether it turned out to be an excellent time to have started practice. People who were returning to London after the war were looking for a doctor, their old GP having moved, or retired, or died. Perhaps, too, those who were still in practice after having weathered the Blitz were overburdened and exhausted and so not too welcoming to newcomers. Also, there was more goodwill surviving from his old practice than he had expected. Between everything the patients came in satisfying numbers. Dr Porter, with whom the informal and unusual collaboration worked very well, guided him in the intricacies of the panel, and advised him also not to accept any patients who lived more than two miles away and none who lived South of the river. By comparison with Dr Clarke-Foster's safaris to outlying suburbs, that policy at first seemed over-restrictive, but, with very few exceptions for more distant patients who lived along quick routes, the Doctor stuck to it, since he realised that, if you were doing contract practice, you could not spend too much time travelling to visit patients. The last quarter of 1946, when his cheque payments totalled £353, and cash takings at the surgery, all duly accounted for, amounted to £15 a week, relieved him of worry about financial progress, and the upward movement continued during the early part of 1947. It was clear that his income would be adequate to pay school fees for the two children, who were now reaching boarding-school age, and to ensure a tolerable life for his wife and himself in a London where you could still go out to eat for a basic 5s. 0d., with fruit, coffee and tips bringing the total to only 8s. 0d. or 9s. 0d. per head. But now, anxiety for the future was even worse. The National Health Service Act had been passed in 1946: the new Service was expected to come into operation in 1948. Should he or should he not go into it?

For those, including doctors who have grown up with the National Health Service, warts and all, it is difficult to realise the trauma which its institution produced in the profession and even, though less violently, in some sections of the public. Long before the war it had been evident to the thoughtful that there must be some kind of change in Britain's system of health care, or rather her lack of a system of health care that covered the whole population. In 1946 the reaction of the British Medical Association, like that of large numbers of individual doctors, suggested that the whole idea of a comprehensive service was new-born, by Beveridge out of Marx.

Dr H. Guy Dain, Chairman of the Council of the British Medical Association, said at the annual meeting in August of that year: 'The principles that are introduced in the Health Bill are State ownership of hospitals, the determination to direct practitioners where they shall not go and prevent them from moving without permission, their remuneration, at least in part, by salary. These are the steps by which it is proposed by the Government that the medical practitioner shall be taken under control in a State service. None of those additions to the scheme will in any way improve the service to the patient.'

This was mild indeed compared with the consort of clarions which sounded from the letter columns of the journal. A Lancashire doctor held that the issue around which the battle waged was 'not health per se . . .; but freedom or bondage. Power-seeking politicians are well aware that complete control of the people, which is essential to their policy, can only be secured by first completely controlling the medical profession . . . Belsens and Buchenwalds are the logical outcome of dictator-made laws when resistance or protests run counter to the whims or fancies of dictator-ministers.'

'Let every doctor then stand firm for freedom and support Dr Dain and the British Medical Association to the limit before the medical profession becomes extinct' cried a voice from Scotland. It stirred echoes further South. 'For nearly 4,000 years the Christlike spirit of our Hippocratic Magna Carta has stood for all that is decent and honourable in our profession. The spirit of that oath has produced a profession which daily performs more for humanity – without thought of gain – than all others put together. In the ultimate analysis, that is the birthright we are asked by a would-be dictator to sell for a mess of Marxian [sic] pottage' (Essex).

'As a learned profession medicine is dead. Practitioners of the future will work a service comparable to the telephone service . . . [he] will choose neither where to live, what type of practice to engage in nor whom to work with. He will be selected for special education at the age of 11 . . . he will not resemble his predecessors in knowledge, interest in his patients or capacity . . . medicine as a profession, as an honoured profession, as a learned profession and as a profession which can offer great help to many friends among the public is dead' (Birmingham).

There were some who supported the proposed new system, and the *British Medical Journal* very fairly published their views, heretical as they must have seemed to the entrenched leaders of the profession. A doctor from Sussex wrote: 'It should be obvious that, however much we may want to retain the right to buy and sell our practices, it is becoming economically impossible to continue the system. How can the average young doctor find, say £7000 capital to pay for his practice, house, furniture and car? And how can he ever pay off a loan from his bank under present rates of taxation? Times are changing and we must adapt ourselves to them.' Another, from Devon, who was among those who had 'looked forward since our student days to a comprehensive health service for the nation' and who 'meant to take part in it if given the honour to do so' complained that he and his fellows were classified 'as "traitors" [Quislings]. Traitors to what? The cause of medicine and the well-being of the people? Or traitors to the interests of Mr . . . [a well-known surgeon] and others like him?' This correspondent went on to make some disobliging comments about 'dishonest doctors who failed to carry out their obligations to their comrades in the Services and who, now being safely established, will not even give them a chance to start again, are now loudest in their protestations against inevitable change', accused the British Medical Association of having already lost a great deal of public sympathy 'by its attitude and its cheap propaganda' and ended by proclaiming 'It is people, not professions, that matter.' A woman doctor from London W6 went so far as to suggest that what one distinguished opponent of the National Health Service 'really' meant to convey by his attack upon it was that 'in future medicine will be no place for a snob, still less for a money-maker'; to quote the *Lancet*: 'The scope for bedside manner and humbug is steadily diminishing.' The *Lancet*, it

123

may be noted in passing, has, in its time, been called: 'The conscience of the medical profession.'

Such enthusiasts were far from typical of the general climate of resentment and suspicion in the profession. Even the teaching hospitals, which received special consideration, approached the new proposals unhappy and mistrustful. Were they not to be robbed of some of their sovereignty and made to accept 15 per cent of women among their students, when most of them had never had any? To the last the British Medical Association fought a rearguard action against the new service which was no less gallant for being, from the first, doomed to failure. Though the general public and probably many doctors may not have been aware of it, the country's medical standards had fallen behind badly since the beginning of the war. The advanced modern treatments would have been beyond the means not only of the poor, but also of those whose resources were modest, and it was clear that there would have to be a broadening of the old insurance scheme to include women and children. Before the war the teaching hospitals had operated on a shoestring. Now they were rather run down, their buildings in many instances needed improvements and they had not got, and in their inmost hearts must have known that they never would get, the money needed to provide for the rapid advances in treatment which were taking place.

The Doctor's worries had nothing to do with the high-minded principles enounced in the *British Medical Journal*, or even with the possibility of the profession's enslavement creating Belsens and Buchenwalds. While he was in India he had decided that he was in favour of a comprehensive health service and now his whole personal inclination was to go into it. He was sure he would have a more relaxed attitude towards his patients if he was not thinking about what he should charge and whether they could afford his visits and if he was giving value for money, and whether they would ever pay him. But what would the nation pay him? Would he be changing a good living for a poor one? Would he lose 'status', whatever that meant and however much it mattered, by going in? Could he be certain of affording public school fees? That peculiarly English obsession, incomprehensible as it is to continental members of the professional classes, was stronger twenty-five years ago than it is today, but even in the allegedly classless society of contemporary Britain, caste marks are so enduring that parents who, principle matching inclination, send their children to state schools may still writhe when they come home saying 'toilet' and 'pardon', then suffer further anguish at their own absurd sensibility to such trivialities.

For the first time in his life the Doctor developed symptoms of a duodenal ulcer, which he kept at bay by drinking quantities of milk three times daily. The situation was not helped by the fact that, while he remained undecided, it was vital that he should build up the practice as quickly as possible, since GPs who signed up for the NHS were to be paid compensation based on their income for the two years before its institution. His earnings during 1947 came to £2,560, but he needed to do better than that, for he still owed £2,500 to his former partner. This was not money outstanding for his original one-third share of the practice: the £4,000 which that had cost had been paid down at the time. But when Dr Clarke-Foster retired in 1941, leaving his young partner to look after the whole practice in wartime London, it had been agreed that the Doctor could buy the remaining two-thirds share for £2,500, instead of the £8,000 which would have been the normal value, and that the sum should be paid after the war. The Doctor finally paid it out of the £6,500 or so which he received in compensation for losing the right to sell the goodwill of his practice when he joined the NHS. The first half of 1948 was reassuring. Cheque payments totalled £1,500, to which was added cash taken at the surgery and carefully accounted for.

On 3 July 1948, two days before the National Health Service came into existence, the British Medical Association, which had at last struck its flag, gave it a muted salute in the editorial columns of the *British Medical Journal*. A state medical service held the dangers of 'dogma, timidity, lack of incentive, administrative hypertrophy, stereotyped procedures and lack of intellectual freedom', wrote the Journal. That was why the medical profession had conducted a vigorous opposition to the variety of White Papers and Bills that had their starting point in the Beveridge Report of 1942. Now 'the doctor will need to exercise much patience and tact in the coming months if his patients demand – as some of them will – the impossible. But with goodwill many of these difficulties will be overcome. The

125

medical man, by his training, has to be ready to adapt himself quickly to new situations, and for this must keep his mind flexible. The Civil Servant, by his training, tends to move with caution and hesitation.'

Adaptability and flexibility are not qualities for which the medical profession is, in fact, renowned outside its own ranks. It might be thought, also, that the use of the word 'training' rather than 'education' was itself an indication that these characteristics were not excessively developed in the generality of doctors.

The same number of the *British Medical Journal* carried a message from the Minister of Health, Aneurin Bevan:

> On July 5, there is no reason why the whole of the doctor-patient relationship should not be freed from what most of us feel should be irrelevant to it, the money factor, the collection of fees, or thinking how to pay fees – an aspect of practice already distasteful to many practitioners . . .
>
> The picture I have always visualised is one, not of 'panel doctoring' for the less well off, not of anything charitable or demeaning, but rather of a nation deciding to make health care easier and more effective by pooling its resources . . .
>
> I know you will be with me in seeing that there does not unintentionally grow up any kind of differentiation between those who use the new arrangements and those who, for any reason of their own, do not.

The Doctor had mixed feelings about Mr Bevan. He thought the Minister had probably been quite right when, having got a broad basis of agreement on the 'new arrangements,' he had fixed a day on which they would come into effect and told the profession to take it or leave it; had he been less decisive the doctors would have gone on nattering for ever. On the other hand, the Doctor thought the Minister had been gratuitously offensive in some of his remarks about the middle classes, and rudeness was never any help in delicate situations.

But he would have underwritten every line of the Minister's message to the profession. In a sense, indeed, he had already underwritten them, for, before July 1948, the Doctor had signed on for the National Health Service. The compensation just about cleared the money he had laid out for his share in his former practice. He was sorry for colleagues who, because of the speed with which the National Health Service had come into being after the end of the war, had had less time to re-establish themselves. Six months after he had joined it, his duodenal symptoms vanished, completely and for ever.

CHAPTER 10

THE APPOINTED DAY:
SOCIALISED MEDICINE
AND WONDER DRUGS

At 9 a.m. on the Appointed Day, 5 July 1948, the Doctor opened the door of his surgery to his first National Health patient. He believed he was, as far as was humanly possible, free of preconceptions about the new service, and he was certain of one thing, you had to begin as you intended to go on. So when, during that morning, a patient who happened to be an MP asked for 500 grains of cascara because he had long been in the habit of taking one every night and it would save trouble if he stocked up, the Doctor had no hesitation in saying no. The National Health Service, he explained, provided only drugs prescribed by doctors, it did not supply or pay for household remedies. The MP was genuinely surprised. He departed saying, though without acrimony, that he intended to raise the matter in the House in order to clarify the situation. He did indeed ask a question, to get a similar reply from the Minister. The MP remained on the Doctor's NHS list until his death, a standing reminder that granting unreasonable, or honestly misconceived, requests was not an essential for keeping one's patients. That early and consistent firmness ensured that the problems with which the Doctor was to be faced during the years ahead never included patients who 'made demands', or 'gave orders'. Neither did he have any personal experience of intentional abuses of the service of the kind which were reported during its early days – 'cotton wool used for stuffing cushions', or 'dressings to make curtains'. In the beginning people sometimes tried to stock the home medicine chest but they were reasonable enough when the situation was explained to them.

There were, of course, difficulties, notably that of numbers. Nobody had really had much idea what the demand would be like at the outset of the new service, though many doctors feared that their surgeries would be besieged. Two months

128

after the establishment of the National Health Service, about 93 per cent of the population had registered with a general practitioner, and the size of the backlog which had piled up over the years surprised even those who might have been expected to anticipate it. The rush for spectacles and false teeth was even more sensational than that for general medical services. Three million pairs of spectacles had been manufactured to meet the demands of the first year: during the first eight weeks, two million went. The amount budgeted for dental services during the first nine months of the National Health Service was £7,150,000. The amount spent was £17,544,783. In all, the first year's costs, which had been estimated at £140 million were exceeded by £68 million.

As for the surgeries, if they were not besieged, they attracted numbers such as many practitioners with experience only of the private sector had never seen or imagined. The Doctor found that, in the beginning, the queues were so long that waiting time (appointments were in the distant future) deterred those who might have been tempted to come with utterly trivial complaints. There remained many with whom, objectively, there was so little wrong that it was difficult not to be irritated unless you could make the imaginative effort of putting yourself in their place. When you did so, you realised that, lacking any medical education or knowledge, you or your wife would have gone to the doctor in exactly the same circumstances. In those early days the Doctor felt that, in spite of a conscious effort to see the situation from the patient's point of view, he sometimes did feel impatient and bad-tempered, chiefly because he had too much to do, but at least, being aware of the danger, he was able to guard against it, hiding his impatience and generally achieving a relaxed consultation. When one had to see a large number of people in a short time it was easy to fall into an abrupt manner, but, quite apart from the human aspect, to do so did not make for efficiency. The patients themselves were often conscious of the queue in the waiting-room, and the sense of pressure tended to make them slower than they would normally have been. If the doctor was feeling the pressure as well, and showed it, he made things worse, and ended by getting nothing out of them.

In controlling his own attitude the Doctor was helped by having seen at first hand how any kind of relationship was damaged when one side despised the other. It had happened in India, when he had frequently been unhappy about the way some Britishers treated Indians. Long afterwards, when reading Leonard Woolf's autobiography, the Doctor was to find a description of exactly that contemptuous irritation with which some doctors regarded their patients at the outset of the National Health Service, perhaps, indeed, still do.

Woolf, writing of his years as a Civil Servant in Ceylon, recalled the time when he had 'sat hour after hour in a kachcheri, watching from his room the perpetual coming and going along the verandah of every kind and condition of human being, transacting with them the most trivial or the most important business, listening to their requests, their lies, their fears, their sorrows, their difficulties and disasters. There are many things in the manners and methods of a Sinhalese or Tamil . . . which are exasperating and distasteful to a European, and many civil servants never really got over this initial annoyance and distrust. However much they liked their work and, up to a point, the people of Ceylon, as they walked into their office in the morning there was below the surface of their minds, when they passed through the crowd on the verandah, a feeling of irritation and contempt.'

What the author was describing was the phenomenon of reaction to suppliants one of whose characteristics was that the irritation increased as people became more suppliant. Woolf had been intelligent enough to recognise it and conquer it. Those who did not risked becoming like the Assistant Superintendent of the police in Jaffna who took the author for a drive in his 'English gig', his conversation interspersed with curses at the drivers of bullock carts who got in his way – ' . . . get out of the light, you black swine' and much else in the same strain. It was the kind of thing that was liable to happen when one's own frustrations and resentments were projected on to the customers.

You had to get above it if you were going to do any good, and the Doctor found that his experience in managing children helped him to do so. Years ago they had taught him that when you wanted to hurry it was often the time to go more slowly. There could be problems also with former private patients, for whom the new service meant adjustments which were often difficult and, sometimes, painful. They had been used to home visits by their doctor virtually on request and to suit their own convenience: some expected to get the same kind of attention, as distinct from the same same kind of medical care, under the new régime. They were deeply offended when they learned that now they were expected to come to the surgery, where they would have to sit in the waiting-room alongside those whom they tended still to think of as 'the great unwashed'. On this point the Doctor was as adamant as he was about supplying drugs on demand. If you were doing contract practice you had to stick to a system of work that was an economic proposition. In surgery one could deal with between six and ten patients in an hour, assuming that they were an ordinary cross-section. It was hard to do more than two or three home visits in that time, and would be impossible when the traffic became thicker. So, clearly, everybody who was not too ill to do so – the Doctor was to prove generous in his interpretation of what constituted 'too ill' – must come to him. Everybody meant everybody, starting with the member of the House of Lords whose wife telephoned to ask if he would come round to give her husband a TAB injection under the National Health Service. Her husband must come to the surgery, said the Doctor. He was too busy to do so, replied the peeress. The Doctor regretted that he also was too busy to visit patients who were well enough to come to him. He did lose those two patients, and a few others like them, while gaining in peace of mind: a quite small number of VIPs, or people who felt they should be treated as such, had a disproportionate nuisance value on a National Health Service list. That list came to include a number of divided families, in which the husband was a private patient while his wife was on the National Health Service, it being supposed that she could spare the time to wait her turn. Sometimes the division was between generations. There were parents who became National Health Service patients while their children remained private ones, on the principle that nothing was too good for them. There were other parents who retained their private status while exposing their children to the Brave New World of the National Health Service – nanny, or, later, the au pair, brought them to the surgery. And there were a few people who came to him as private patients to see the form and, having decided it was OK, changed to the National Health Service. The Doctor found this as infuriating as did most of his colleagues; one felt that one had been taken for a ride.

He gave up his anaesthetic sessions at Tite Street after about six months of National Health Service work, hearing as he did so the echo of Dr Clarke-Foster's voice. One of the maxims of his old principal had been that fixed appointments like hospital and clinic sessions did not fit in with general practice, where you already had to make fixed consulting times for surgery. If you added to them you would not be free enough to visit patients or to respond to a really urgent call. In order to be clear for his hospital sessions the Doctor was doing some calls between 8 and 9 a.m. and finishing the less urgent between 9 and 11 p.m. It was not good enough either for his patients or himself, but that was only one of the reasons which impelled him to give up when he did. He realised, perhaps a little earlier than some of his colleagues, that anaesthesia was becoming, if it had not already become, a specialty in its own right, rather than a pleasant side-line for GPs. His own training at St Thomas's, when each student was required to give twenty anaesthetics, had been followed by very considerable experience as a Casualty Officer at the hospital, at Tite Street before the war, and as an anaesthetist in private practice, but he could not claim the specialised training and experience which was becoming increasingly necessary as more sophisticated materials and equipment came into use. So he stopped both the hospital sessions and private bookings, which had anyway been decreasing because there were fewer nursing homes, and found that the loss of the £400 from Tite Street was not reflected in his annual income.

It was a tough year and, at the end of it, there seemed little reason to suppose that the future would be any less tough, but there were some things to be counted on the credit side. Looking back, he could not see that his relationships with his patients had in any way deteriorated because they no longer paid him directly, discounting those few with whom he had parted company. There were some with whom it had improved because the Doctor felt more relaxed about visiting them now that he no longer had to count the cost in cash. From the bread and butter standpoint, it was already clear that, under the National Health Service, it was possible for a GP to make as good a living as he would have done in private practice unless he was one of the small group who were out-standingly successful. One's income was steady and predict-able, one was spared those ghastly accounting sessions every quarter and the new system seemed to him remarkably free of form-filling. True, you were required to keep record cards for your patients, but a competent practitioner was already doing that. It was an opinion which the Doctor was never to have reason to change. In so far as the clerical work of the practice did later increase, it was because there was a gradual improve-ment in communication between hospitals and GPs, who got, however belatedly, full reports on the treatment which their patients had received.

There was an unlinked factor which irradiated the sheer slogging of those early days: while the National Health Service was accomplishing its social revolution, antibiotics were revolutionising medicine. For patients the date which counts is not that on which the discovery of a 'miracle cure' fills the headlines, but that on which it becomes generally avail-able. The gap is variable and can be considerable. The dis-covery of Prontosil, the forerunner of sulphonamides, had been announced in 1935 and, as we have seen, well before the war the Doctor had his first experience of the therapeutic power of those red tablets. Prontosil was an effective drug in itself; as early as 1936 it began to cut the death rate in puerperal fever, which was then about 1,000 a year. In 1938 it was supplemented by the sulphonamides, notably the famous M and B 693, which trans-formed the treatment of pneumonia. By contrast, though the spores of penicillin had drifted in through the window of a labo-ratory in St Mary's Hospital as early as 1929, it was not until 1940 that it was standardised and its therapeutic powers an-nounced, and not until after the Second World War that it was available for all patients who needed it.

In that first period, administering penicillin was a compli-cated business. The drug was not stable in water, so that a new solution had to be made for each injection. Since injec-tions had to be given at four-hourly intervals, day and night, it was extremely difficult to use outside hospitals or nursing homes, unless a patient had round-the-clock nursing care at home. To overcome this handicap penicillin was put up in wax, which was just sufficiently fluid to be injected and, since it was absorbed more slowly, needed to be given only twice a day. In the icy bedrooms which were common at that period it was extremely difficult to handle, since, in winter, the whole ampoule became solid and had to be warmed slowly in hot water. When it did reach a liquid state it cooled so rapidly that injections were made possible only by the use of a needle with a very wide bore, so that it could be drawn up into the syringe before it solidified once more, and a wide-bore needle made the procedure even more unpleasant for the patient. In the late 1940s a doctor would set out on his rounds with his bag weighed down with a battery of sterile glass syringes – disposable plastics were a boon of the future – wide-bore and otherwise, which it was often necessary to re-sterilise before the end of the day. Boiling was the only available method of sterilisation, outside institutions that were equipped with autoclaves. It had the extra disadvantage that, fairly soon, either the glass barrel of the syringe or the metal plunger became slightly distorted by the heat so that the fit was no longer precise and part of the contents leaked back past the plunger and never got into the patient. It tended to leak also over the hands of district nurses who were called in to give injections to patients being treated at home. This was the cause of some of the cases of penicillin sensitivity which became evident in the late 1940s. Another was the introduction of penicillin ointment for infective skin conditions: there were few quicker ways of developing an allergy to the drug than having it put on your skin every day for a week or so. The immediate rash was a minor nuisance: more serious was the possibility that people so sensitised might collapse if they were given a penicillin injection and, if they were not within reach of modern methods of resuscitation, might die. As more refined forms of the drug were developed, allergy became less common. At worst, it had to be seen against the enormous benefits of penicillin, which cured most pneumonias – until its advent, the existence of viral pneumonias, as distinct from bacterial, had scarcely been recognised – and it reduced enormously the incidence of mastoid infections.

Its very effectiveness made the infections which it did not touch, TB, all viruses and children's infectious diseases, stand out more clearly. There came the discovery also that, even in its own field, it had limitations. Before the end of the 1940s some germs achieved immunity to it, but as this was becoming dangerously apparent, new antibiotics appeared. Tetracyclin proved capable of doing some things which penicillin could not, such as helping in the cure of viral pneumonias. Streptomycin, used in conjunction with other drugs, was so successful against pulmonary TB that what had been a lingering, very often fatal disease became a readily curable illness. Chloramphenicol, which, from the start, could be given by mouth, had a direct effect on whooping cough at a time when vaccination against it was not particularly efficient, but had to be used with great circumspection as it could do damage to the blood which was sometimes irreversible. Typhoid and typhus, in the treatment of which it is of special value, are rare in this country.

When they had behind them generations of virtual helplessness in face of disease, it is easy to understand that, at first, doctors could scarcely believe in this sequence of miracles. Shortly before retiring, the Doctor talked to a man who had been his patient for twenty years, and learned for the first time that, in 1946, he had had acute osteomyelitis, or infection of the marrow of the bone. In hospital he was told of the seriousness of his condition; doctors discussed the possibility of amputating a leg, but finally treated him with penicillin. In doing so they warned him that, while the new drug would defeat the infection, he was likely to be left with some disability, and the prognosis for his being able to walk in the future was gloomy. Twenty-four years later he was still walking without the slightest trace of handicap.

There was similar incredulity about the possibilities of streptomycin when it began to be used against tuberculous meningitis. It was a disease which had had an implacable 100 per cent mortality. The Doctor who, as a young physician at Tite Street, had been moved by the tragic case of the baby who had been infected by its father on week-end leave from a sanatorium, had seen one in his own practice shortly after the war. The patient was a girl of fourteen, suffering from scarlet fever, whom he had treated with either penicillin or one of the sulpha drugs. The scarlet fever improved, but the child's condition deteriorated so sharply that she had to be admitted to hospital. There she was found to have generalised TB with meningitis which had been activated by the infection. Only two or three years later he had another case, a boy of sixteen

135

or seventeen, in whom the disease had a fairly acute onset. The Doctor got him into hospital at once and he was treated early and energetically with streptomycin. He recovered completely, with no after-effects whatsoever: nevertheless, when he reached call-up age he was turned down for National Service because he had once had TB meningitis – it was not yet recognised generally that total cure with no residual brain damage was possible.

The cost of these daily miracles was astronomic, in the sight both of doctors, who were used to buying pills at 5s. or 10s. per hundred or even per thousand, and of patients, who had grown up with the idea that a bottle of medicine cost 1s. 6d. or half a crown and lasted a week. Injections, when they were necessary, had always been more expensive. In the old days Dr Clarke-Foster had charged 7s. 6d. for giving an injection, over and above the cost of the material, a practice which the Doctor did not continue after the war. But when penicillin was first introduced, the amount needed for a single injection cost about 15s. 0d.; a tablet of tetracyclin or chloramphenicol cost 2s. 6d. and one had to swallow eight in a day. In reality, as the Doctor fairly soon came to realise, from the patient's point of view it was a good bargain because, before the war, a serious illness inevitably meant a formidable doctor's bill. He remembered, during the 1930s, sending a bill for £90 to a man who had had an attack of streptococcal pneumonia which had kept him in a nursing home for three months, during a fortnight of which the Doctor had visited him twice daily. It had seemed a shocking sum to have to find. Had tetracyclin existed at that time, the patient would have had to swallow two tablets every four hours for five days, and then he would have been about cured. Half a dozen visits from the doctor would have brought the total of £13 16s. 0d. compared with £90. It was difficult to get private patients to see the situation like that; they continued to be thunderstruck by their chemists' bills.

For doctors, even the most disabused, 'bliss was it in that dawn to be alive', though the sense of wonder soon faded into an acceptance of the commonplace. Its memory did not fade; on the threshold of retirement the Doctor could still recall vividly the stimulation of that time when, at last, one could defeat infections against which, previously, one could do so little. Inevitably the unaccustomed sense of power had an intoxicating effect. For a time, actively encouraged by the pharmaceutical companies, doctors tended to think that every new treatment was going to be as effective as penicillin and tetracyclin. Many of the new antibiotics had, indeed, considerable value, but as supporters only. How was a busy practitioner to steer a course among the multitude of new drugs, or of new presentations of the same drug – Prontosil, a crude sulphonamide, was at one time on the market under seventy different proprietary names – which would combine safety with the best use of new discoveries? It was a question which was to be asked more urgently after the thalidomide tragedy, without producing any very conclusive answer. The Doctor gave fervent thanks that he was not involved in it, while realising that he might well have been, for Distaval, the proprietary name under which the product was marketed in Britain was, in ordinary use, an extremely useful sedative which had looked like being very valuable indeed.

With hindsight he felt that, in common with large numbers of his colleagues, he had had a period when the first excitement and delight in being able at last really to do something was followed by near-blind faith in the virtue and potency of the new drugs; but, relatively, he regained a degree of critical vision fairly soon. When amphetamines, in the form of Dexedrine, had been introduced in the 1930s, he had prescribed them for patients suffering from low blood pressure, but had suspected that the seeming improvement they produced was little more than amphetamine euphoria. After the war he used Dexedrine for depressive states, but gave up prescribing it very early, when he found that students were taking it before examinations, and examiners said they could distinguish which students were under its influence because they wrote repetitive rubbish but came out of the examination highly pleased with themselves. It was true that, when combined with barbiturates in the form of 'purple hearts', under the proprietary name of Drinamyl, it was, in certain instances, a successful symptomatic treatment, but it was one to which patients became rapidly and permanently habituated. He was left with three whom he was unable to wean from it. Fortunately they were responsible individuals, who were able to keep to the very small dose to which they were accustomed; it did no harm to their health and it did give them a certain uplift, which they needed. There were, however, many cases of irresponsible people increasing dosage, which did great damage.

The Doctor was cautious from the start about steroids, more generally known as cortisone. British hospitals did not use them for some time after they had been introduced in the USA and, like penicillin, they were not at first available on general prescription. When they did become available, they seemed to promise the answer to two ills for which GPs had long been searching for a remedy, asthma and rheumatoid arthritis; but the potential danger of their side-effects was so considerable that the Doctor soon decided that a wise and careful physician in general practice should avoid them unless they were the only possible remedy, and would in no case use them in the long term without having the treatment started in hospital after assessment. It was a policy which was to earn him an abusive letter from the husband of a patient whom, in conjuction with the Senior Physician of a teaching hospital, he had treated conservatively, with no great success, for persistent back pain and depression. She emigrated to the USA, where, since fashions in these things vary from country to country, she was given cortisone. The spectacular effects inspired her husband's letter to the Doctor, whom he upbraided for not himself having had the sense to use it. The Doctor would have been interested to know the permanent effects; he knew of many patients who had later had cause to regret their treatment, but there was no follow-up letter from the indignant husband. He stuck to his policy, using cortisone on his own initiative only to cut short attacks of asthma, and even here there were difficulties. Used externally, usually in the form of hydrocortisone ointment or lotion, it made an enormous difference to the control of eczema and allied skin conditions.

However credulous doctors may have been in the aftermath of a break-through which was as epoch-making as the discovery of antiseptics or X-rays, or the development of anaesthesia, it was on the public that the antibiotic revolution left the most permanent mark. From now on they felt, and have largely continued to feel, that there was a magic pill for any condition. In reflective moments the Doctor sometimes wondered if there was a link, however remote, between that dawn

138

of an age of faith, twenty-five years ago, and the present wave of drug habituation.

CHAPTER 11

FIVE YEARS' HARD:
SHOULDERING THE LOAD

If, towards the end of his career, the Doctor had been asked which period of his working life he had found the most demanding and taxing, though not necessarily the least rewarding, he would have had little hesitation in settling for the first five years of the National Health Service. During that time the new service displayed in their most acute form all the problems which were to be endemic within it, from trouble about pay, which led general practitioners to the brink of a strike, to a shortage of hospital beds for the elderly which caused some of them to spend their last days in conditions which were deeply shaming to a supposedly civilised country. The background was a tempo of work which made the average GP feel that each year consisted of twelve 'flu-ridden Februaries. The Doctor emerged from it all with his interest in his patients intact, with his techniques for combating unhelpful officialdom greatly reinforced and, even more important, with a clear idea of the function of a general practitioner working in a health service in an era of increasingly specialised medicine.

The pay dispute was only one aspect of the financial difficulties which were to dog a service which had been undercapitalised from the start. Two facts which were evident to the Doctor from a very early stage were that the cost of the NHS had been grossly underestimated and that some, at least, of its teething troubles were due to the fact that there had been no attempt to educate the public in the proper use of this new benefit. When those who, previously, had had medical attention only if they were seriously ill, and sometimes not then, were told repeatedly that now they, too, had a right to the services of a properly qualified doctor, it was hardly surprising that some of them should bring their coughs and colds and minor aches and pains to the surgery. They were behaving as a large section of the upper and middle classes always had behaved. On balance, the Doctor was surprised at how moderate the public were in their demands. If they had woken up to what they could get and come and got it there would soon have been a state not of financial difficulty but of financial crisis.

As it was, perhaps the first of the several disputes over earnings between the medical profession and the government, which took place in 1957, should be ranked as a crisis. When the NHS was established, the rates of pay of GPs and specialists respectively had been decided by two committees, each presided over by Sir Will Spens. The rate was set by establishing an average for the earnings of various doctors before the war, and, if necessary, adjusting them to what the committee considered an adequate level for that period. For GPs Spens came up with a 1939 figure of £1,111 a year. It was for the government to interpret that sum in terms of post-war money values, also to take into account possible changes in earnings in other professions. The government, too, devised the method of payment, which seemed almost deliberately tortuous. All the capitation fees for all patients were put into a pool, which was then divided between all the doctors who were providing general medical services, according to the number of patients on their lists. Since there were some deductions from the pool for temporary patients, fees for anaesthetics and the like, and since more doctors were liable to come in during the course of the year, the amount received by each executive council at the beginning of it was always less than in fact it spent, and it could be another twelve to eighteen months before the accounts for any one year were finally wound up. The difficulties involved in administering the estates of doctors who died did not bear thinking about: proving a will must have taken up to a year and a half. Probably the doctors felt from the first that the Government had set the current equivalant of 1939 values too low. By 1951 continued inflation, linked with the complexities of the system of payment and the unremitting workload, drove them to threats of a strike. Finally the dispute went to arbitration and in the following year the High Court Judge, Mr Justice Danckwerts, who heard the case, decreed that the current equivalent of Spens's 1939 figure of £1,111 should be £2,222.

The award was backdated so that the amount involved was

substantial; the Doctor's share was £1,800 which, even after half of it had been paid back in income tax, was quite a powerful shot in the arm financially. But he had worried a good deal while the BMA was talking about strike action. By temperament the Doctor was so strongly opposed to violence that he felt striking was justified only if one was in actual want, and that a strike of doctors, which meant inevitably that their patients would be regarded as the bargaining counters, was profoundly unethical. Did the fact that he worried mean that he was afraid that, in spite of his convictions, professional solidarity might involve him in the movement? certainly, when, during the 1960s, general practitioners came even nearer to the brink of a strike, the Doctor showed no signs of worry, having decided that professional solidarity must bow before individual conscience. He would have felt that he was losing his soul if he had joined in the strike, and there is little doubt that he would have gone on working even if he had been the only GP in London of the same mind. He was asked at the time if there were any circumstances in which he would strike, and said yes – the threat or existence of clinical direction. He was careful to define his terms: clinical direction meant being forbidden to prescribe for NHS patients any drug which he might prescribe with benefit for private patients.

The National Health Service did, from the start, exercise some financial control over prescribing, in addition to laying down the general principle that, if the same drug was available both in a proprietary brand and in the supposedly equivalent standard form, a practitioner was expected to choose the less expensive. It is questionable whether practitioners invariably do so, chiefly because not all accept the theory that the two forms are equivalent. In addition to this, an average was established for the prescribing costs of GPs in every region. Anybody who exceeded it by more than 25 per cent was required to give an explanation, and if this was not satisfactory, part of his remuneration was withheld. The Doctor thought this a crude method of costing, unless the authorities took into account the methods of treatment of every doctor and the length of time his patients were off work. His own handling of 'the English disease', chronic bronchitis, provided an illustration. Since the advent of antibiotics he had educated the sufferers on his list into an entirely new attitude towards their illness. Traditionally, they had soldiered on as long as possible until they had to take to their beds, the attacks becoming progressively worse and more frequent as time went on. It seemed extravagant to keep them on prophylactic doses of antibiotic, at £2-£3 per week, throughout the winter, but if one took lost working time into account, it was cheaper in the long run, apart from the fact that the sufferers lived longer and better. In consequence, the Doctor's prescribing costs were consistently higher than the local average but he was never required to account for them, which suggests perhaps that the 25 per cent margin was adequate to cover the kind of active policy he adopted.

By contrast, there seemed nothing to be said for the prescription charges, originally set at one shilling, which the government introduced in 1951. They led Aneurin Bevan to resign, and were opposed even by the BMA until 1964, in which year the annual conference of the association did a right-about-turn and decided to support the charges because of their 'deterrent' effect. The Doctor detested them when they were introduced, and continued to detest them up to his retirement. He deprecated the principle of a tax on the sick, and he thought it outrageous that dispensing practitioners should be required to collect the shillings which patients, not unnaturally, often thought were going into their doctor's pocket. Had the Doctor done his own dispensing that situation would have been far more likely to make him withdraw from the NHS than inadequate pay. Finally, when the charges were first introduced, there was no agreement whether a prescription was to be defined as a piece of paper or as each separate item which was written on it. In haste it was decided that it was the paper, with the result that doctors wrote even more illegibly than usual, in an effort to get everything on to a single sheet.

Those things were details, however irritating. The difficulty of getting elderly patients into hospital was an acute problem whose consequences could be tragic. It was one to which the character of the Doctor's new practice made him peculiarly sensitive. Having started it from zero in 1946, he had had about 2,500 patients when the NHS was established. By the beginning of 1951 he had 3,600 on his list, which was 100 more than the recommended maximum. During his years in practice in the same area before the war the Doctor had thought he had come to know the local community; now he realised that he had known only a section of it, those who could afford to pay something for their medical attention, and so were not dependent on the 'parish doctor', a practitioner who contracted with the local Poor Law authorities to look after the indigent.

Now, a large number of the very poor, most of whom were also the very old, came on to the Doctor's list, and during the monthly visits which he paid to those who were housebound, whether or not they were being treated for some specific condition, he learnt the worst about their living conditions. The majority existed in the basements of terraced cottages or in single rooms high up in nineteenth-century blocks of flats, or in houses let off in warrens, where water came from a cold tap on the landing and the lavatory might be three flights down. At this level the equivalent of the two elderly sisters who had spent their days at the Army & Navy Stores was an old lady living in a terraced cottage not a hundred yards from the Doctor's surgery, who, all day, sat on the edge of her bed wearing nothing but a nightdress, contemplating a half-full chamber pot. Periodically neighbours brought her food, part of which she scattered on the floor to feed the mice who were her only friends. Should she not have been in hospital, or, better, in an old people's home? The Doctor was not certain that she should, since what she dreaded most was being taken away from her home, miserable as it was, but the question was in any case academic, since there would have been at the time no hope of getting her into either. He saved his efforts for cases like that of a solitary old man living in a building belonging to the Metropolitan Association for Improving the Dwellings of the Industrious Classes, whom he found helpless in bed, incontinent, filthy, and suffering from bronchopneumonia and malnutrition; or another, living in an old, low-rent block of flats, who was discovered collapsed and immobile. Left at home, he would have been condemned to lie in his own excreta for hours. Hospitals had no bed for either, at a first request. It was the winter when there were attested cases of old people's having been put out into the street while somebody telephoned an accident ambulance which would take them to hospital as casualties. Once in, one might hope they would be allowed to stay. The Doctor never resorted to those tactics: he

144

doubted if he could have done so with a quiet conscience. His campaign on behalf of his own patients was carried on by means of persistent telephone calls to all who might possibly be concerned, letters to the influential who might have a string to pull, and newspaper publicity when occasion offered.

The Doctor found an old friend to back him up. Mr French, of the City Council's Public Health Department, had survived the Blitz and was now applying his talents to the social problems of peace; to which he brought the same good humour and resource that he had shown in tackling the problems of an air-raid shelter. His talents included a useful gift for bending regulations up to, but never beyond, the point of fracture. The Doctor made also a new friend (who was a very similar character to Mr French) while at the same time completing the education in public health medicine, neglected at St Thomas's, which had begun for him when, as a young practitioner, he had done sessions at the ante-natal clinics of Heston and Isleworth. Now, through a professional contact with Dr Andrew Shinnie, Westminster's Medical Officer of Health, which developed into a personal friendship, he began to understand its human side and to realise the potential of an intelligent co-operation between GP and local health authority. In the years to come he was to be increasingly grateful for the many physical aids for his elderly or handicapped and housebound patients which had formerly been supplied through hospitals and which he could now obtain from the local authority simply by signing a chit – wheel chairs, walking frames, handrails beside baths, ramps over steps, virtually any existing equipment which made it possible for sufferers to keep their independence. True, there could sometimes be an inordinate time-lag between request and delivery, but the Doctor was an assiduous and generally effective prodder-into-action in such cases. It was Dr Shinnie who was largely responsible for the initial help and continuing support which Westminster gave to the local branch of the National Old People's Welfare Committee (now Age Concern), the voluntary organisation which had been founded in 1940. The Doctor was soon a member of the local committee, feeling that, in post-war conditions, he could do more useful work there than on the Westminster Housing Association.

Immediately, the two public services which were a revelation to him were home helps and home nursing (the latter was not to become a local authority responsibility until early in the 1960s), closely followed by meals-on-wheels. The home help service, in fact, dated from before the war, but at that time had been used almost exclusively by women who were confined at home and were not able to make any other arrangements for keeping their households going. Its great expansion after the war was chiefly for the benefit of the old and infirm, and the Doctor came to have an enormous respect for the real devotion of many of the women who worked in it. They often did more than they were asked, providing a friendship and interest, sometimes involving their husbands and families, which was even more valuable than the household cleaning which was ostensibly their job. There could be problems, which the Doctor was often called upon to sort out, whether by persuading a proud and independent old lady that she would not be accepting charity if she consented to have a home help, then further persuading her not to work herself to the point of collapse over cleaning the house ready for the help's arrival, or in acting as a buffer between a possibly confused old person and an indignant home help whom she had accused of theft. The last was a peculiarly difficult situation because, in the nature of things, it was impossible to establish the truth. Even nurses were sometimes accused of theft, though rarely; but, in his experience, doctors never. They, instead, were charged with poisoning the patient or making her worse. Each to his trade. . . . Tricky as they might be to resolve at the time, those difficulties were trivial compared with the benefit received by large numbers of frail old people who were enabled to continue living in their own homes by the props of a home help, a meal service, and visits from a district nurse. The Doctor was never able to fathom the reasoning which decreed that the first two should stop at week-ends and over holidays like Christmas and Easter, when they were needed more acutely than ever – so badly, indeed, that some home helps paid unofficial visits out of the kindness of their hearts. Was it supposed that the old did not eat at week-ends, or did the authorities subscribe to the myth that all had loving relatives who would materialise on Saturdays and Sundays to feed and cherish them?

District nurses never stopped, and the Doctor, who had pre-viously had no first-hand experience of their work, was unbounded in his admiration for it. He had, of course, always known of the existence of the Queen's Institute of District Nursing, and of the reputation it enjoyed, but, before the war, he and Dr Clarke-Foster had looked upon it as a service for the near-indigent, not for the paying patients who had made up their practice. For the more modest end of it they had used an independent nurse and midwife, both of whom became the Doctor's patients after their retirement, and remained with him until they died.

If more prosperous patients required full-time nursing in their own homes, they called on the excellent agency in St George's Square, run by Mrs Coward, aunt of Sir Noël, the quality and experience of whose nurses was guaranteed as far as was humanly possible. Only in reasonably substantial households was a patient able to be looked after in that way, for the private nurses, who found much of their employment in home confinements, expected to be waited on, with dining-room meals brought upstairs. They would undertake no cook-ing beyond heating milk or making tea, and even that not in the kitchen. If a house did not provide services of that kind the patient had to go into a nursing home. Revolution came after the war, when, following a period of two or three years during which nursing homes and agency nurses were equally scarce, nurses from Australia and New Zealand came to work in London, usually as a means of financing their travels in Europe. They were attractive, intelligent, well-trained young women who, though they did not expect to be hired as cooks, were quite prepared to do anything to make life go easily in the household which employed them. But for the most part they did not live in, so that twenty-four-hour care involved three nurses working eight-hour shifts, whereas, under the old system, one nurse had covered the whole day and another the whole night.

The district nurses, particularly the permanent staff nurses of the Queen's Institute, maintained a standard whose dedi-cated efficiency was in the best St Thomas's style, than which the Doctor knew no higher compliment. It was more than a matter of first-class bedside nursing. So often a severe illness could mean a degree of chaos in a household, with more or less well-intentioned neighbours doing nothing very effective. The advent of the district nurse seemed to settle everything; organisation and relief came in with her. Normally, communication between GP and district nurse was effected by means of the message pad which the latter left at the patient's house, on which she wrote details of injections, dressings and so on, and he wrote any necessary instructions. Sometimes the Doctor used to make an appointment to meet the district nurse at the house of a patient, usually in cases where there were extensive dressings which he needed to see.

Soon, he found himself lecturing district nurses at Islington, and another group in Bloomsbury, about doctor-nurse co-operation. He was interested to notice that no district nurse ever told a patient her name, though, inevitably, patients often got to know it. Was it so that there would not be requests for particular individuals? The Doctor inclined rather to the idea that, like the custom of referring to St Thomas's Sisters by the names of their wards, which helped to discourage an undue familiarity between Sisters and doctors or students, it was a legacy from Florence Nightingale. According to her canon, the nurse was less a woman than a beneficent presence, without body, parts or passions. In the climate of the mid-nineteenth century, only by establishing that principle would it have been possible to recruit young girls of good family into the nursing profession. Up till then, its public image had been pretty accurately typified by Dickens's Sairey Gamp, unjust as that portrait undoubtedly was to many of the conscientious women who were the ward sisters of the period.

As for himself, while the Doctor was human enough to wish that the working day was not quite so long, nor so close-packed, he never for a moment felt that, in this greatly changed system, general practice was being devalued, or that he was losing his 'real doctoring' to the hospital. True, the hospital gained more prominence in the perspective of the average practitioner because now, at least in theory, the diagnostic aids of its laboratories were available to him. GPs had long had access to the bacteriology provided by the local authorities, but this seldom went beyond public health needs, like examining throat swabs for suspected diphtheria, or sputum testing for TB. All other chemical or bacteriological investigations had to be entrusted to private pathologists, unless a GP was in a position to get it done at his own teaching hospital by means of the old-boy line. Two or three years after the NHS was established, one could apply, particularly in London, to hospital laboratories for a fairly wide range of investigations, though the teaching hospitals lagged behind the old local authority hospitals. If only unofficially, there was some limitation on the service, which was confined to the quicker and cheaper investigations; for anything more elaborate the patient had to be sent to Outpatients, where, in the Doctor's experience, the physician who examined him came to exactly the same conclusion as he had done himself, and he had to wait a month for the answer. The Doctor thought this tiresome and time-wasting, just as he thought grossly wasteful of manpower the lack of any service for collecting specimens, which meant that a doctor might spend forty-five minutes a day being his own errand boy.

It was partly because of that state of affairs that he developed what was to be his continuing attitude to hospitals and consultants, namely, to think of them as technicians. They were often brilliant technicians, besides being extremely careful and conscientious. There were certain patients whom the Doctor referred to them – without having kept exact figures he would have put the proportion at somewhere between 10 and 20 per cent, most of them psychiatric cases – about whom he was in real doubt and difficulty, needing and getting a great deal of help in their treatment. With the great majority he knew perfectly well what operation was indicated, or what investigation was needed to prove or disprove his diagnosis; he referred them to Outpatients so that the physician or surgeon could arrange for it. His own job was to prepare the mind of the patient in advance; to explain that hospital appointments could not always be precisely timed, since a physician or surgeon who was both teaching students and examining patients could not know in advance how long he would spend on each case; to interpret the consultant's advice, sometimes even to convince a patient that the hospital and the consultant really did know what they were about. There was no question of 'handing over' his patients; he was their doctor, and so long as he was interested in them, and showed it, there would never be any danger that he would lose their respect.

His own role, he realized, had changed from what it had been when he started in practice in 1933. Shortly after giving up anaesthetics, and for much the same reasons, he had given up midwifery. Surrounded as he was by teaching hospitals, all with students and midwives with their tongues hanging out waiting for maternity cases, he would not have got a sufficient number to maintain his skill. Also the NHS arrangements for maternity, which did not require the GP who assumed responsibility to be in at the delivery, was not his idea of looking after a patient. He gave up, too, nearly all minor surgery. For a GP in a country district it was no doubt still a necessary part of the job; in Central London it was not.

What it amounted to was leaving to the hospital what it could do better than he could, and himself doing what it could not do at all, which was looking after the whole patient. Diagnostic skill was more vital than ever when so many people, suffering from such a variety of ills of body or mind, presented themselves daily at the surgery. Continuing care was almost equally important, so was visiting a fair number of them in their own homes, for how else could one gain a real understanding of them? Patients needed somebody they could count on, who would be there from start to finish, not contracting out when they were guilty of unacceptable behaviour such as not responding to treatment: somebody who would be unfailingly on their side, an Ombudsman to whom they could turn when they were bewildered by incomprehensible or inflexible official regulations.

Practising what the Doctor, who was not much of a one for modish jargon, never learned to call the 'holistic approach' was a demanding job, but it had its rewards. Sometimes he was made aware of them in unexpected ways, as when, passing through the courtyard of a block of council flats, he would hear one of a group of pre-school-age children say: 'That's my doctor!' and others chime in to claim possession also. They and their parents were his patients in a way they would not have been in pre-war conditions, when you could never be sure that households who called you in for measles might not call in somebody else for mumps. Now, as long ago in a hospital ward, the Doctor knew those for whom he was responsible, and felt himself to be part of the community as he had never been before.

CHAPTER 12

NEW DEVELOPMENTS:
HARDWARE AND SOFTWARE

When, in 1946, the Doctor restarted in practice in Dr Porter's first-floor front, it would still have been possible to say that he was running a cottage industry. He was single-handed and he had no ancillary aids, though almost immediately he began to employ a part-time secretary who fairly soon became full time. When, towards the end of the 1960s, he was approaching retirement, it was as the principal of a four-handed partnership which had a district nurse and psychiatric social worker attached, employed four secretary-receptionists and ran an appointments system. The story of the evolution of the one into the other was highly typical of the development of general practice during those years.

Like the vast majority of the period, the practice premises were not purpose-built. The fair-sized Victorian house in which the Doctor had occupied the first floor and Dr Porter the ground had originally incorporated the dwelling and surgery of an elderly practitioner of thrifty habit. Because a street-lamp shone directly into the master bedroom, which, during the next ownership, was to be used as a consulting-room, he had seen no necessity to have it wired for electricity. Dr Porter's original partner, when he took it over, made good the deficiency. The Doctor, in his turn, had water laid on. Getting rid of the nuisance of having to go up or down a flight of stairs every time he wanted to wash his hands was worth the £50 it cost to pipe in a supply and install a hand basin and geyser.

Neither he nor Dr Porter had any hesitation in replying no when, in the early days of the National Health Service, the Medical Officer of Health for Westminster had asked practitioners in the area if they would be interested in taking premises in a local authority health centre; and they suspected that they were two among many. Health centres

151

had been included in the original concept of the NHS, though the Doctor doubted whether all concerned were sure that they meant the same thing by a health centre. To GPs at that time they meant above all the possibility of control of the way they did their work, and they fought shy of an innovation that seemed to threaten the independence which, for many, was what had led them to choose general practice.

From the start the Doctor's unofficial and rather unorthodox association with Dr Porter worked well: the two alternated on week-end duty and stood in for each other during holidays. Their compatibility made them the more conscious of the precariousness of the arrangement. If one were to die or move, the local Executive Council, without consulting the other, could fill the gap with any candidate it wished. Partners, by contrast, could themselves appoint a successor to a vacancy, or choose a new colleague to enlarge the firm. In 1951, accordingly, the two regularised their position by entering into a formal deed of partnership. Immediately the practice increased in value because NHS payments were designed to encourage partnerships by an appropriate loading of capitation fees. Numbers of patients were increasing also, at a rate which made it practicable to appoint a third partner. It was not an ideal number for arranging night or week-end cover; they solved the problem by inviting a woman doctor who ran a single-handed practice near by to join their duty rota, which ensured three clear nights and three week-ends out of four for each of its members. When their woman colleague retired in 1966 the partnership had increased to four, so that it was able to operate a self-contained rota, except for employing a locum, who was usually a Registrar from one of the neighbouring teaching hospitals, to take one daily surgery during the holiday period.

The Emergency Call Service, a deputising system by which, on payment of a fee, practitioners could have their night calls referred to a central agency which was in constant radio contact with a number of duty doctors in cars, was introduced in the mid-1950s. Fifteen years later, 65 per cent of the GPs in Inner London used it at times. The Doctor and his partners were not to be among them. They had no reason to doubt the efficiency of the service, what they questioned was the ethics of handing over a patient to a doctor whom one did not know

152

and whom one was never likely to meet.

Nor did they fuse their practices when they formed the partnership. Each partner conducted his individual practice in his individual consulting-room, which, they felt, helped to personalise the relationship between the patient and his own doctor. The fact that all the consulting-rooms were under the same roof made it easy for the partners to pool their experience, but there was no question of a patient's having to see whichever doctor happened to be on duty when he or she came to the surgery. All held their daily surgeries at the same time; other than at night or at week-ends it was only in a situation of rather unusual urgency that a patient would see a doctor with whom he was not registered, and even then there was a probability that he would be familiar at least by sight. Soon the three partners were employing two secretaries between them, and early in the 1950s they consulted an architect on the possibility of adapting the surgery premises so as to provide a reception area instead of perpetuating the situation by which patients walked in from the street to their doctor's waiting-room. It proved impossible, short of turning the caretakers out of the basement and the top floor, since there was no land for building an extension. That factor was limiting the physical improvement of a great many town practices in the early years of the NHS. At the time the Doctor and his partners did not seriously consider starting an appointments system. The minimum cost would have been another full-time secretary-receptionist and an extra telephone line, with no financial return for the outlay. Payment by capitation fees with the same standard allowance for practice expenses, whether a doctor spent anything on improvements and equipment or not, did not encourage lavishness in such matters.

So the surgery queues went on and moves towards greater efficiency in the organisation of the practice were more modest. Each partner established a weekly session for children's inoculations, and by the mid-1950s all had acquired a dictaphone or a tape-recorder for their correspondence, so freeing for visiting a part of the normal working day which would otherwise have been spent dictating to a secretary. All three, also, began to pay a small salary to their wives for answering the telephone at home – it was not until near the end of the Doctor's career that the setting up of an efficient central call service in London enabled thousands of doctors' wives to obtain a divorce by mutual consent from their husbands' practices. The NHS made no allowance for this, the only benefit was a certain income tax relief.

In spite of the difficulties, practice improvement was in the air; it was to be one of the twin themes which dominated a couple of decades, the other, necessarily linked, being the long war over remuneration waged between the BMA and the Ministry. At last, probably inspired originally by the war rather than the NHS, medical administration and organisation was beginning to blossom in the hospitals. They started to send out regular typewritten précis on patients, which, in their turn, made practitioners more conscious of the importance of record-keeping. The Doctor had kept records almost from the first, having early decided that, even if he had thought Dr Clarke-Foster's system, or lack of it, was a wise example to follow, his memory was not good enough to allow him to do so. Those who were convinced that, far from being phased out in an area of scientific medicine, general practice had a vitally important part to play in the medical care of the future found encouragement and continued support for their belief in the setting up of the College of General Practitioners, which, within a few years, was to become a Royal College. The Doctor was in touch with the beginning of this development and he was one of the 1,077 founder-members – from a total of about 22,000 practitioners who joined within three weeks of the launching of the college in 1953. Had time allowed it is likely that he would have been as deeply involved as were two or three of his old Cambridge contemporaries, but time limited extraneous activities severely, particularly if one aspired to have any sort of family life.

Work, by now, had settled to the rhythm which was to continue, virtually unabated, until the time of his retirement. He saw from ten to fifteen patients at morning surgery and from fifteen to twenty-five, at worst, thirty, in the evening. Home visits varied from about a dozen to twenty a day, and only if patients chanced to live near one another could one hope to do more than three an hour. This meant that, most evenings, there were from two to half a dozen visits still outstanding after evening surgery. He fitted some in between 7 and 8 p.m., before supper, and more often than not, at least in winter, went out again after it. He got home soon after 10 p.m. to dictate on to a tape-recorder the letters which his secretary would type on the following day.

With such a time-table, it is perhaps a little surprising that he should have said that doctors had 'always been prone to build up a myth that their work was harder, more taxing, more strenuous than anybody else's'. He did not subscribe to this, believing that a business man who took seriously both his job and his place in the community had no more spare time than a doctor, and knowing from observation that journalists and people in television or show business had far worse hours than doctors. He added that he had himself been obliged to work at full stretch in order to ensure his future, because his first twelve years in the profession had been totally unproductive of savings and, since he could hope for no more than twenty or twenty-five years of NHS practice, he would receive less than the maximum pension.

The Doctor quickly realised the importance not only of organising one's work efficiently, but of avoiding, or, at any rate, trying to avoid, being frightened by its sheer mass. The only way to cope with a heavy load was to plod on as efficiently and as quickly as you could without seeming to hurry, until you got to the end. The important thing was to satisfy your patients, and very few people could do that if they were giving out an aura of hurry and bustle. Satisfied patients were not 'demanding'; it was the anxious and those who felt, sometimes, perhaps, with reason, that their doctor had fobbed them off hastily, who made demands and turned up at the surgery more often than their physical condition would seem to warrant.

The way to satisfy patients was to let them see that, during a consultation, they had the whole of your attention and interest, and that, if they needed reassurance, it was given only after a proper examination. Once you had won – and earned – their confidence it was unlikely that patients would become demanding and over-dependent. There was some outside evidence that the Doctor managed to cling to these principles even in circumstances which might have presented the temptation to abandon them. 'I do hope he won't bother to examine me tonight – I'm in a hurry' said a new patient one evening, when the waiting-room was crowded and the surgery

155

was running late. There was more than one supporter for the voice which replied: 'If he thinks you want examining, you'll get examined, never mind if it's ten o'clock at night. He's thorough.

The Doctor found that his ceiling for surgery patients was ten an hour, which did not mean that he spent six minutes with each. An average group was likely to contain two or three patients who wanted a repeat prescription, perhaps for a chronic condition, or certification for a few more days' convalescence. From them one made up the time for those who needed, and got, a good deal longer than six minutes. A January day on which he saw fourteen patients during a two-hour surgery, spending forty minutes with the first and fifteen with the last, was not altogether typical because, as a rule, he made special times for those patients, often suffering from depression, or some other form of mild mental illness, who were likely to need longer than fifteen minutes, but it was typical of the flexibility of his approach. As in the old days at the Victoria Hospital for Children, he found that time given to a patient at a first consultation was more than regained during successive ones.

There was an order of precedence, also, for home visits. It was an absolute rule of the practice that if a patient requested a visit it was made on the same day, unless the caller was able to be convincingly clear that the matter was not urgent. First visits were made during the morning, repeat visits during the latter part of the afternoon, the period immediately after lunch being devoted to special appointments. In theory his regular visits to elderly patients also were made during the afternoons; in practice they often had to be fitted in after evening surgery. When there was a rush of work those monthly maintenance visits could be used as a buffer against the pressure. The elderly soon learned that 'See you in a month's time' did not necessarily mean four weeks to the day. But see them he did, even if it sometimes meant visiting during what should have been a free week-end. He knew it was a bad thing to cut into your time off but there were occasions when it could not be avoided.

Unlike some GPs of the period, the Doctor and his partners never attempted to reduce the load by putting up a stiff resistance to visits. Apart from any humanitarian aspects, it could be dangerous. Sooner or later one was virtually bound to come across a patient who was unable to put across on the telephone the urgency of the need, and then one would be on the road to disaster. It was particularly important to respond promptly when the patient was a child, in whom a feverish state might be the beginning of almost anything. Here many a late evening call ensured an unbroken night for a doctor, since a promptly administered antibiotic would take effect before midnight. It was risky also to follow the example of certain practitioners who never went back once a patient had been put on an antibiotic. No doubt the habit reduced their visiting list most satisfactorily, but an antibiotic did not always work. One had to see for oneself that it was working and then decide, according to the circumstances of the case, how many return visits to pay.

Night calls, in the Doctor's experience, were not a serious problem. He would almost have been prepared to say that, from the patient's point of view, they were hardly ever unreasonable, though a large number turned out to be not medically necessary. But, reasonable or not, they did require a good deal of self-control in a doctor, who had to be sufficiently on the ball to sense the need of a frightened, unhappy caller when, understandably, he felt cross and sleepy. It might have struck a blow for the medical body politic if he had given even shorter shrift than he did to the young woman who telephoned at 1 a.m. to ask the time of morning surgery, but it would have been terrible if he had given a cruel, or even brusque, answer to the one who rang at 2 a.m. to say she thought her son was dying. The Doctor went with all speed, to find a perfectly healthy, though bewildered, boy of fourteen, wrapped in blankets, propped up in a chair with his feet on another, while his mother hovered over him anxiously. When she had got up to look at him she had thought he had stopped breathing, she told the Doctor. After telling the boy to remake his bed and get back into it, he stayed long enough to discover that, a short time before, the mother had woken to find her husband dead of a coronary beside her. She, of course, was the patient. Treatment was organised later on the same day, and she never put through another 'unreasonable' call.

Besides his NHS list, the Doctor, like his partners, had a small private practice, which all regarded as providing a little jam to their bread. The Doctor's argument in favour of the continued existence of a certain amount of private practice was not that a state monopoly was even more undesirable in medicine than in other departments of life, but that a private sector would act as an exemplar and pacemaker which would stimulate generally higher standards. All told, he estimated that he devoted the equivalent of two hours a day to private work, which meant something more, and more varied, than seeing private patients. One of the most rewarding – the word is not used in its strictly financial sense – of those outside jobs was a renewed association with the industrial firm which, during the Blitz, had asked the Doctor first to inoculate its staff against tetanus and typhoid and later to hold a weekly surgery for those who, because of the bombs or the black-out, found it difficult to get to their own doctor after work. Now he did two weekly sessions which, since the timing was fairly elastic, did not clash with the demands of his own practice, and which soon proved to have a greater content of welfare than of medicine – not that the Doctor would have found it easy to draw a firm line between the two. Since those he saw all had their own doctors in their home districts he would in any case not have felt justified in treating any other than minor conditions, and even then, on occasion, he was careful to let the patients' own doctors know what he was doing.

It is worth noting that he did not undervalue the welfare content of these sessions as being 'not real medicine'. On the contrary, he enjoyed the work, finding it relaxed, and worth while, and a bit different. The Royal Society of Health invited him to carry out medical examinations of new members of the staff, which was no more interesting than any other routine medical examination, but it led to a pleasant association with the RSH. Acting as medical adviser to the Royal National Lifeboat Institution was far from routine; the duties ranged from holiday visits to crews in the Hebrides or the West of Ireland to testing equipment for keeping survivors warm, in the garden on a frosty night in January, with committee work in between. For the Doctor, as for many of his colleagues, the possibility of such interests, some of which might be ranked as professional hobbies, would always be among the attractions of general practice.

The extraneous activities included a development which

was one of the twin landmarks of the 1960s. The Doctor had always maintained contact with his old teaching hospital, practising as he did virtually in its shadow, and gained from it valuable help and support, and opportunities for learning of new developments in medicine which served almost as a continual if informal refresher course. In 1958 he had been invited to deliver the annual Lecture on General Practice, which was virtually the only attention that St Thomas's, in common with most other teaching hospitals, then gave to the subject. Times have since changed, but between the original neglect and the present serious teaching of the subject in the Department of Clinical Epidemiology and Social Medicine, which includes studying the medical needs of a community in the field, there was an interim period of two or three years during which the Doctor lectured students on general practice, with emphasis on its social medicine aspect.

The medical care of students had remained what it was when the Doctor himself had been one. If you felt ill you consulted an appropriate member of the staff, choosing your moment as seemed most suitable, for there were not normally any fixed times for such consultations. It was not an ideal system, chiefly because it made no provision for dealing with the depressions and problems to which students in general are acknowledged to be liable, and which, in medical students in particular, are apt to be exacerbated by the phase of hypochondria almost inseparable from the study of medicine, when the pupil is convinced that he is suffering from one or more of the diseases about which he is learning. As a result, students were often left to try to contain a good deal of anxiety, with varying success. When, during the 1960s, it was decided that there should be a student health service, one of its aims was that it should give some help in these situations. Evidently the Dean of the Medical School, R. W. Nevin, who had been one of the Doctor's students when the latter was Dr Cassidy's House Physician, and his colleagues did not share the opinion of Lord Moran that GPs were doctors who had 'fallen off the ladder' of professional advancement, for they wanted the new service to be run by 'real' GPs, who were practising in the outside world as well as in the hospital community, and the Doctor was asked if he and his partners would start it.

Besides being understandably flattered in human terms,

159

they were interested and stimulated. Here was the ideal link between hospital and practitioner. The Doctor had always been doubtful of the real value to a GP of holding an appointment at a town hospital, which was a very different proposition from working in a cottage hospital in the country. There could, of course, be exceptions; before many years had passed one of his own partners was to be running a dyslexia clinic at St Thomas's purely because he had gained expertise in a little-known disorder which was recognised as being the cause of some of the reading difficulties suffered by children. But more often than not a clinical assistantship for a GP meant tagging on to a consultant, doing nothing very significant. Here they would be appointed as clinical assistants who were paid by the medical school, who went into the hospital to do their own job and who would have the opportunity of doing it in the best possible conditions. They had full backing from the hospital laboratories, X-ray facilities and consultants and, if they thought it desirable, could refer their patients to consultants outside the hospital. Also, which was almost equally valuable, they could use the consultants' dining-room. This was not just a status symbol. It established, as it was intended to do, easy two-way communication between consultant and GP, which is rare now that it is only during a domiciliary consultation that the latter is likely to be present when his patient is seen by the former. Indirectly also, though perhaps at this stage neither the Doctor nor his partners framed the idea very clearly, the new scheme might influence the idea which students had of general practice. As things were, and as they had been in the Doctor's time as a student, their impressions of a whole branch of medicine could be unfavourably coloured by two or three mediocre doctors practising near a teaching hospital and referring to it large numbers of patients with dubious diagnoses and deplorable letters.

The extra workload involved taking on a new partner, bringing the strength of the firm up to four. All had been St Thomas's students, and three were linked with the hospital by family connections or through marriage. One, the convent wall by now having fallen, had married a Nightingale. They had no feeling of being strangers in unfamiliar surroundings when they got the scheme off the ground in 1965.

At about the same time came a happening which led to the

transformation of their home practice. In 1965 the Ministry of Health had introduced an improvement grants scheme which repaid to doctors one-third of the cost of improving their premises. In 1966 the 'New Deal' for doctors provided for the reimbursement of the rent and rates of surgery premises and of 70 per cent of the salaries of ancillary staff. At the time, the first was of no interest to the partners, who had established more than ten years earlier that they had no possible space on which to improve. Suddenly a single-storey building next to the surgery house fell vacant, and they snapped it up. Once more the architects were called in, and, this time, they came up with a scheme for a reception area with waiting-room, an office and four consulting-rooms. There were manifold delays before the conversion was completed, and there was also the discovery that the Ministry of Health had abandoned the original policy of letting GPs have, for improving their premises, the compensation which was due to them for their surrender in 1948 of their right to sell the goodwill of their practices. The Doctor and the senior of his three partners – Dr Porter had retired a few years earlier – had thought of using this to fill the gap between the improvement grant of £1,500 and the total cost of the conversion. When they learned that the Ministry would not hand over the capital, on which it was paying interest at $2\frac{3}{4}$ per cent, but was prepared to lend the necessary sum at an interest of $7\frac{3}{4}$ per cent, they decided to make other arrangements. The end of 1967 saw the job finished.

An extra secretary-receptionist was taken on, and the practice began 1968 with an appointment system. Just short of twenty years after the establishment of the NHS the hardware had caught up with the soft, to use the terminology of the computers, which, the Doctor fervently hoped, would remain the servants of medicine and not become its masters.

Attachments of local authority staff, which are usual, if not universal, in group practices, did not lag far behind. All four partners, who were unanimous in their admiration for the work of the district nurses, were delighted to have 'their own', whom they saw daily, and to whom they could give instructions about patients, or exchange information, instead of scribbling notes to each other, or making what were inevitably chancy appointments at the bedside of a patient.

In theory the Doctor was greatly in favour of the attachment of a psychiatric social worker, since he was conscious that a considerable number of patients on his list who were suffering from psychiatric illnesses could benefit from the support of somebody who had more time than he was able to give them. Unfortunately, as he thought, it was arranged that the PSW, instead of paying follow-up visits in their own homes to patients who had seen the doctor at the surgery, should herself hold regular surgery sessions. It was a doubling which neither side found particularly satisfactory, and the PSW was later withdrawn.

No health visitor was attached, which was regrettable if only from the standpoint of the Doctor's continuing education. Like many GPs of his generation he was in his inmost heart probably less convinced of the value of health visitors than of that of district nurses. This is due partly to the fear lurking in the mind of a professional that another professional may be giving contrary advice to one of his patients behind his back. It is an attitude which is easier to understand if one remembers that this is how health visitors sometimes feel about doctors. Additionally, older doctors did not meet health visitors during their training in the way that they met nurses. They were not quite sure what the health visitor did, and at the back of the minds of many was a phrase about 'the nurse who never takes her coat off'. At least the Doctor made an effort to overcome his reservations. Before his retirement he was ready to agree that somebody who combined the functions of health visitor and medical social worker would be of great value in the practice. Among other contributions she could take over some of his regular maintenance visits to the elderly, though, most emphatically, not all of them. Perhaps two visits out of three. They were his patients and his concept of looking after them did not include handing over their care even to the most competent and devoted of ancillaries.

CHAPTER 13

PROBLEMS: PRESENT, PROSPECTIVE, PERENNIAL

It was some time during the 1960s that the Doctor, in conversation with a friend, said there seemed to him to be less and less difference between being a doctor and being a priest, except that, as a doctor, you got more money.

You got a good deal more, and the public seemed to feel it right that this should be so. In 1955-6 the average – median, not mean – income of all NHS doctors was £2,300 a year; for consultants it was £3,130, for GPs £2,160. In 1957, shortly after the Royal Commission on Doctors' and Dentists' Remuneration had begun its three-year labours, the *Lancet* indulged what some of the rearguard of the medical profession regard as its Quisling tendencies by conducting its own survey of public ideas about, and attitudes to, the earnings of doctors. The survey revealed that doctors' pay was consistently under-estimated, both absolutely and relatively to that of other professions, and that its comparative economic worth was rated highly. More than half those questioned thought doctors earned less than £2,000, one-third that they earned less than £1,500 a year, and only one in forty over-estimated their earnings. Even among the better educated, only half knew that doctors earned more than MPs, but two-thirds thought that they should do so, while very few thought that the clergy should get more money than they did. Perhaps the most striking indication that this was a newly anointed priesthood was the belief of more than three-quarters of the survey that if doctors left the NHS, as they had threatened to do, they would still see all patients, charging only those who could afford to pay. The *Lancet*, if only by implication, was a little caustic about this simple faith.

The Doctor's remark was prompted less by an awareness that he and his colleagues had been chosen to bear the virtues of the world than by experience with his patients who, increasingly often, brought to him problems which were not strictly medical, in the sense that some of them, while they certainly affected health, could have been handled equally well by a wise and experienced priest. Were there more problems nowadays, or fewer wise and experienced priests, or was it simply that, particularly in towns, people were losing contact with any form of organised religion, even when they were not losing all religious faith? The last certainly; at the same time they were manifesting a sometimes very primitive faith in 'science', a term which embraced most things from antibiotics to psychology, as the answer to all their troubles. It may have been, too, that the Doctor attracted rather more confidences and appeals from the worried and the near-desperate than some of his colleagues, if only because of his readiness to listen. He was accepting, receptive and as non-directive as was humanly possible. The more self-aware of his patients came to rely on him as a touchstone by which they could restore a temporarily disturbed sense of perspective. 'I can't imagine any situation in which one would go to him and say: "I know you'll think I'm silly, but . . ." ' said one of them. He never did think people were silly, or rather, he accepted that all humanity is silly at times. The less articulate, in whose vocabulary phrases like 'the value of catharsis' did not figure, came away after a surgery session feeling that, if only for a time, the load had been lightened. According to the circumstances of the individual case, there might or might not be a prescription; there were patients who felt that, when there was, it was not always the most valuable factor in the treatment.

Along with the problems brought by their patients, and an aggravation, sometimes a dramatic one, of those which had always existed in general practice, like drug addiction, mental illness and the care of solitary old people, doctors during the 1960s were faced with certain problems different in kind from those of the past. Within a relatively short space of time a practitioner who had adjusted to the situation produced by the Pill had had to make up his mind about abortion, and could scarcely help realising that, before very long, he would have to decide his attitude towards euthanasia.

During the Doctor's student days contraception had not been in the curriculum; consequently, like the great majority of practitioners of his generation, he had not given advice in methods of birth control, referring patients who asked for it, or for whom it seemed indicated, to one of the doctors who specialised in the subject. Almost all had been middle-class patients, for the wives of weekly wage-earners had gone to the clinics run by the Family Planning Association. The FPA did not give advice to single women, so teenage girls, if their partner was not using a sheath, simply hoped for the best. The coming of the Pill brought them all to the surgery, since they needed a prescription for it, and brought also the inevitable wave of antagonism from the righteous, who were either sincerely horrified at what they considered to be a fall in standards of public morality or simply jealous that everything was being made easy for the young women of today. It was never quite as easy as was publicly supposed: the Pill disagreed with some women and the threat of thrombosis, which was the basic problem, remained. About its effects on public morality the Doctor was less ready to pronounce. There was little doubt that it led to more extra-marital sex, but a good deal of it was between partners with a solid relationship, which often matured into marriage, whereas previously the same couple might have married when the girl became pregnant, with less happy results. Certainly the availability of the Pill lowered the age for sex and that in itself could present difficulties. What did you do as a family doctor when a girl of sixteen, whom you had known from infancy, came to the surgery asking to be put on the Pill? It was a situation which the Doctor never ceased to find sad, and the conflict of loyalties between the girl and her parents could be painful. But he believed that if the girl was over the age of consent she had as much right to expect absolute confidentiality from her doctor as had any other patient. Never, in such a case, did he tell the parents what was going on, but never, either, did he give a prescription for the Pill without a preliminary discussion in which there was no element of condemnation on his side. He doubted if it ever had the slightest effect on any girl's decision, which would have been firmly taken before she came to him, but at least it left the door open for her to return for help if things went wrong.

The evolution of the Doctor's attitude towards abortion typified that of public opinion in being a gradual conversion from the total opposition, unless the life of the mother was directly endangered, which had been the line at St Thomas's during his student days, to the belief that, more often than not, it was the lesser of two evils. 'Respectable' abortion had, of course, existed long before the Abortion Act 1967 made it legal to terminate a pregnancy for social and psychological as well as physical reasons, long, also, before the famous 'Aleck Bourne case' brought the matter into the open in 1938 (Aleck Bourne, a well-known gynaecologist, terminated the pregnancy of a young girl who had been subjected to multiple rape, then admitted having done so, in effect saying to the authorities: 'What are you going to do now?' His trial and acquittal, even if it had little effect on current practice, made the public give thought to a matter which, until then, they had managed to disregard.) For fifty pounds it was possible to get an abortion done in a nursing home by a properly qualified surgeon. At the other end of the scale was the back-street abortionist, with her knitting needle or syringe and her doses of gin and penny royal. The fees here were from £3 to £5; the results, which were often dreadful and sometimes fatal, were liable to bring the patient into hospital as an emergency.

After the war, but before the Act, the resistance of hospitals to performing abortions lessened: psychological as well as physical reasons might be admitted, and many GPs who were not themselves opposed on religious grounds had a list of liberal-minded gynaecologists among whom they 'shopped around' for the benefit of their patients. Consultants tended to be more sympathetic towards middle-class than towards working-class girls, presumably because they found it easier to identify and sympathise with them. Even after the Act was passed, the Doctor found that the attitude persisted in some hospitals. Apart from that most flagrant kind of injustice, he could see no logical basis for any sort of discrimination between one request and another now that the procedure was legal – finding the necessary hospital accommodation and staff was another matter. There was a perfectly clear case to be made for forbidding abortion unless a continued pregnancy would threaten the life of the mother, but once it was liberalised, then every woman should have an equal right to it. By that he did not imply what is sometimes called an 'on demand service', but that all requests should be sympathetically considered. The decision whether or not to have her child must rest with the woman herself, but before taking it she should be given a chance to discuss the situation with a counsellor, and, in taking it, she should be protected against pressure from parents and relatives. Since the counselling should involve after-care, the Doctor thought it would usually be better done by the woman's GP, but there should be an alternative, as some practitioners would not want to undertake the task.

The Doctor followed that policy in his own practice, taking every girl and woman who asked for an abortion over the pros and cons of the situation as impartially as possible. None the less, of all the duties which fall to a general practitioner, managing an unmarried pregnancy, whether it was aborted or came to term, was the one he liked least. Whatever the solution adopted, it almost invariably involved a tragedy for somebody, and there were so many of them that, after a time, he was able to sense what a girl had come to see him about almost as soon as she was inside the consulting-room door. Sometimes she was afraid to tell her parents, being convinced that they would turn her out; then a doctor who knew and was accepted by both sides might be able to serve as a bridge between them. Sometimes her parents already knew, and it was they who were virtually insisting on an abortion. Almost without exception the girl herself wanted to have and to keep her baby, and to look after it herself. In an ideal world the Doctor was convinced that that would be the best solution for a single woman: in the existing world it was seldom practicable. There were working-class families who might cheerfully accept an illegitimate child, but he never knew this to happen in a middle-class family. The next best solution was adoption, with the shortest possible period of fostering intervening. All too often the actual alternatives were abortion or the likelihood that a child would spend its formative years in conditions which offered little hope for its future stability and happiness, and, when a third life was at risk, abortion seemed the lesser wrong. In his experience it almost invariably left the young mother with a burden of guilt and a longing to know what the child she did not have would have grown up into.

The advocates of the Abortion Bill had made much of the needs of married women who found the task of looking after their existing families almost more than they could cope with or the means of the household support, but during the whole of his time in practice the Doctor was only twice approached with a request for an abortion by a married woman. The first came from a woman who had just lost her husband and felt that she could not go through with her pregnancy. For once the Doctor's side of the discussion which followed was rather heavily loaded: he let it be seen that he thought she would do well to have her baby. She had it, and was permanently grateful for having been encouraged to do so. The second was from a woman already the mother of two children, and slightly depressed. The Doctor had not thought hers a very strong case for abortion – it was before the Act – but had nevertheless referred her to a hospital, where it was refused. The child was born and grew up on equal terms with its two elders in what was a comparatively prosperous family, and the mother suffered no ill effects, but the Doctor was certain that, ten years later, she would still have said she would have preferred an abortion. It was difficult to argue anything from two such disparate cases. In the meantime, now that abortion was legal, the Doctor wished that some of the people engaged in the clinic business would stop behaving as if it was not. They gave no aftercare, and, in contrast to NHS hospitals, never sent him, as the patient's GP, any details of the case. The women themselves tended to believe that there could be no complications after so simple a procedure. All too frequently there were; if they were seldom dangerous to life, they could affect health and future fertility.

Since he believed abortion to be right in certain circumstances, and even believed that it might be justifiable to end the life of a dreadfully deformed child within half an hour of its birth, he found some difficulty himself in understanding the grounds for his total opposition to euthanasia. If one accepted that life began at the moment of conception, what was the moral difference between terminating a pregnancy and ending a life which seemed to have become a burden? He decided that, for him, the question turned on whether what one was extinguishing was human life or a human being who had had experience of life. A newly born infant had had experiences only in the uterus and during the process of birth; to the Doctor neither could be counted as 'experience of life'. He distinguished, also, between euthanasia and so-called 'mercy killing', believing that this if only rarely, might be justified, though should never be admitted as a recognised procedure.

168

Neither did his scruples prevent him from giving maximum relief of pain, even when doing so involved the risk of shortening a patient's life.

But nothing could persuade him that the existence of a legal and formalised procedure for committing murder was compatible with the protection of the individual, or see euthanasia as anything other than a euphemism for a Hitlerian disposal of sub-standard humanity. Not only was it repugnant, there were practical difficulties. Its advocates usually had in mind two separate groups of people. The first was made up of supposedly well-balanced individuals suffering from a painful and incurable illness who took a deliberate decision to have their lives ended, though not by their own hand. During all his time in practice, the Doctor had never known anybody who would have taken such a decision. Many people when they were gravely ill had phases of wishing they were dead, but that was a far different thing from going through a legal process whose object was permitting somebody else to murder you. He had known one or two terminal patients who had killed themselves, but he doubted whether they would have been considered sufficiently well-balanced to sign a document. He had known also a few who would have taken this decision in order to relieve relatives of more distress – sometimes those relatives were exercising an influence on the patient. That, the Doctor thought, was not a good enough reason.

The second group were those who, from age or disease, had been reduced to a vegetable existence in which they were not capable of deciding or signing anything at all. Many were being lovingly and competently cared for by relatives. Who was to apply for euthanasia? Was it to be the doctor or the relatives? Certainly not the doctor, or not the doctor who was looking after the patient. Perhaps there might be a visiting specialist who went round signing death warrants. It could be the relatives, but, if it was, the majority would feel guilty for the rest of their lives. That would leave a few who would be only too glad, or who had been impatiently waiting to inherit, which suggested that if euthanasia ever became legal there should be a proviso that all property involved should go to the state, not to the patient's family or medical attendant.

Far more important than euthanasia, in the Doctor's view,

was the need to upgrade geriatrics and to improve the quality of terminal care, whether in hospital or at home. There was no logical, ethical or any other justification for allowing the senile indigent to end their days in third-class hospitals. Technical equipment in such hospitals need not be anything like so elaborate as in acute hospitals, nor staffing so highly specialised, but standards of care and comfort should be equal. They were not, partly because geriatric hospitals had developed from the old workhouse infirmaries, and inherited their tradition, partly because of the factor which, from the start, had dogged the extension of the social services, the belief held by a section of the public, and encouraged when it had not been implanted by certain MPs, that once people started getting something for nothing there would be no end to it, and the aged would be clamouring for admission to their three-star hospitals. The Doctor doubted it: in his experience, the aged, like most other people, greatly preferred their own homes, however decrepit, to any kind of hospital.

In acute hospitals, now that treatment was so much more possible, he suspected that effort was sometimes put into hauling patients back from the brink of the grave by increasingly ingenious methods of resuscitation which would have been better spent in helping them to move tranquilly towards it. There were circumstances when 'officiously to keep alive' was neither wise nor kind. True, the problems which cropped up were not always as straightforward as they could be made to sound. If a patient in the last stages of a painful illness developed pneumonia the first instinct of a doctor might be to say: 'Thank God!' and not use an antibiotic. If one could be sure that the pneumonia would be fatal, many doctors would be glad to let it follow its course. But suppose, instead of killing the patient, the pneumonia were to develop into pleurisy, which would add further distress and discomfort to the remaining weeks of his life?

The fact that, by the very nature of their work, teaching hospitals, where medical students got their training, were not places in which one learned anything much about terminal care meant that it was seldom particularly well managed in practice either, except by a fairly small number of older, experienced GPs, some of whom were extremely good at it. It was true that a system of payment by capitation fees did not encourage the frequent visiting which could be of such immense comfort to the patient and his family. But was there also a kind of arrogance, or perhaps a kind of cowardice, which made doctors 'lose interest' in patients who were not going to recover? And how great must be the peril of both for consultants who, generally speaking, were in at the death only by accident, and whose patients, again generally speaking, had moved out of their aura before grave deterioration was apparent. Perhaps it would be a good thing if somebody endowed a Chair of Easeful Death at one of the more forward-looking universities . . .

The post-war wave of drug addiction did not make a serious impact on the Doctor's practice: partly because addicts, particularly young ones, usually avoided ordinary GPs; partly because, by one of the odd quirks of the human geography of Central London, the practice area, which could show a generous share of human frailties and aberrations, including the more florid, had no great concentration of addicts. Before the war, in Britain, drugs of addiction were limited almost entirely to morphine, with some chloral – heroin was extremely rare – and addicts were popularly believed to be those who had easy access to supplies, doctors, nurses and veterinary surgeons. Such cases as came the Doctor's way confirmed that idea. Teaching hospitals virtually ignored the subject, merely pointing to the existence of the problem as a warning of the danger of keeping patients on morphine for too long a period. The Doctor could not remember ever having been taught how to manage addiction: he doubted, indeed, whether, at that period, many consultants knew any more about it than that it was dangerous to withdraw a drug suddenly, and suspected that most would have regarded addicts as being beyond the pale and refused to handle them. Somewhere he did glean the information that cannabis, as well as morphine, was widely used in the Far East, and that Orientals were less severely affected than Westerners, as they did not continually increase the dose. When the war took him to the Far East he was able to check it against the existing situation. Several members of an Indian unit attached to HQ in Ceylon were receiving a daily issue of opium and, upon inquiry, the Doctor found that, in certain parts of India, addiction was so widespread that, if it had not been forthcoming, there would have been a catastrophic fall in recruiting. So the British Raj had been gently blackmailed into organising supplies for those who were registered as opium-eaters. There was no discernible effect upon their health or efficiency, which suggested that the East had indeed adjusted its social behaviour to the recognition and use of certain drugs, as the West had done to its own drug of addiction, which was alcohol. That, in the West, was respected and respectable, firmly entrenched between social customs and vast vested interests, and so long established that many people were able to use and enjoy it without dangerous consequences – the Doctor was among them. But anyone who doubted that it was an addiction had only to look back at what had happened in the USA, when Prohibition was introduced, to see a continent behaving collectively like an addict.

In common with all other practitioners the Doctor had among his patients a number of unhappy drop-outs whose drinking had caused them to lose jobs, health and their place in the community, along with more who were half-way along the same road. Not all were men, but the pattern for women was different. Their drinking was so secretive as, on occasion, to deceive even themselves. He had had as patients women who believed sincerely that cider, Campari and medicinal tonic wines were all innocent, even when taken in large quantities. Statistics were not a reliable guide to the consequences of alcoholism: if only out of consideration for the relatives, few doctors, when making out certificates, would give drink as the cause of death, true as it might be, directly or indirectly. It was because he had seen all too often the cost in health, domestic happiness and working efficiency of excessive drinking that the Doctor was absolutely against the free sale of cannabis, believing that our society could not afford another drug whose effects, in the long term, might be worse than those of alcohol. He was not sanguine about the prospects of treatment for any kind of addiction. In his experience, dependence on a drug was a sign of immaturity, or of psychiatric instability, which came to much the same thing. He was convinced that, for either condition, the most hopeful remedy was not therapy in adult life, whose results were seldom brilliant, but changes in education and in living patterns which would enable more children to grow up successfully without craving the stimulation or sedation of a harmful drug. There was one kind of alcoholism in which the sufferer had long 'dry' periods, with lapses which were almost always triggered off by recurrent attacks of depression. For the depression there was effective treatment, but almost invariably the patient turned to the bottle to find relief from his misery, instead of coming to the surgery at an early stage.

To be strictly logical, smoking, which was as addictive and enjoyable as thumb-sucking, for which it was the adult substitute, should be included among harmful drugs. Even if research, financed by manufacturers apprehensive about their sales, succeeded in isolating and removing the carcinogenic elements from tobacco, the smoke would still act as a lung irritant, so that over-indulgence was a sure way to contract chronic bronchitis. The Doctor sometimes thought that the people who devised warnings about the dangers of smoking were on the wrong track. Real and hideous as was the possibility of lung cancer, a betting man would say that the odds against a heavy smoker getting it were favourable. There were no odds at all against the same smoker, in his later years, being severely handicapped by bronchitis – it was a dead cert.

Mental illness, by contrast, was far more in evidence in the practice than it had been before the war, when, broadly speaking, it had been limited to 'breakdowns' for the educated classes and compulsory certification for the rest. The Doctor would have found it hard to decide whether what is vaguely known as 'modern life' had really been responsible for an enormous increase in depression since the time when he first entered the practice, or whether it was just that, on the one hand, doctors had learned to recognise it, and on the other, the gradual evolution of more sympathetic public attitudes, together with the discovery of drugs which gave relief, meant that sufferers were less likely to hide their troubles and had more encouragement to bring them to the surgery. What without doubt did increase steeply after the passing of the Mental Health Act, 1959, which put mental illness on the same legal footing as physical illness by encouraging informal entry to mental hospitals and early discharge from them, was the number of mentally unstable patients in the community. It was probably true that the policy of early discharge was responsible for an increase in the number of vagrants sleeping rough and unable to fit into society, but the Doctor, whose thinking on quite a few social matters had a refreshing streak of unorthodoxy, was not sure that this mattered greatly. Better that they should be free and vagrant than kept in hospital and permanently institutionalised. If there were too many vagrants the public might become conscious that mental hospitals were omitting to prepare the ground adequately before discharging patients, and so, by degrees, there might be some improvement. Pending it, one could do something to help those who came to the surgery; given time, one could have done a good deal more. Schizophrenics as well as depressives clearly got considerable relief by coming to the surgery to talk in the knowledge that their ideas, however bizarre, would provoke no reaction of shock or disapproval, and, in the case of the latter, that they would not be told to pull themselves together.

There was no lack, now, of more tangible means of relieving symptoms and controlling conditions. Towards the end of the Doctor's time in practice there were more than eighty proprietary drugs listed in the pharmaceutical indices as sedatives and tranquillisers, and forty as anti-depressants, all new since the war. Having selected that or those which suited the individual patient, and, so far as possible, ensured that he took his tablets regularly, the vital point was to be sure that he was not taking anything else as well. In combination with some of the new drugs even simple household remedies which patients had for years been prescribing for themselves could be dangerous: the last twenty years had produced a whole set of problems relating to reaction to drugs, singly or in combination. It may be noted that the Doctor spoke and thought of the 120-odd psychotropic drugs in the armoury as 'relieving', or 'controlling', not as curing. Only when it was known how much so-called 'mental' illness was due to metabolic change in the body rather than to a basic fault of the central nervous system could treatment be as precisely aimed as was that of so many physical ills.

There remained the perennial problem of general practice, the situation of solitary old people. 'Modern life' had certainly intensified it, though, in the Doctor's view, far less by weakening the sense of family responsibility, as was sometimes suggested, than by breaking up natural communities. When son and daughter-in-law were living in a Midlands industrial

174

town, and grandchildren were at university in the North, worlds away in more than one sense, was it to be wondered that a grandmother left alone in a one-room flat in Central London should begin to withdraw from the world? It was true that, compared with the days when the Doctor started in practice, there were far more agencies which tried to keep such people as far as possible in the normal stream of everyday life, and there were many of the elderly, lonely and possibly a little shy, but not natural solitaries, whose lives could be virtually transformed by their efforts. But there were others who lived by and on their ferociously indomitable independence; if, with the best of intentions, welfare workers overcame it and took them to a home where they would be well looked after but totally dependent, their spirit was broken and they lost the will to live. Sometimes it was possible to catch them at the beginning of the cycle of growing inefficiency and eccentricity which normally led to total isolation and, it might be, to a solitary death from undernourishment and deadly cold. At that early stage, by infinite patience, somebody might succeed in gaining the confidence of one of these isolates and becoming his link with the world, indeed with life itself. The Doctor had himself managed it in a few cases: he shared with a local psychiatric social worker the distinction of being one of the only two visitors against whom an embattled old lady did not use the broomstick which she kept behind the door to repel all comers. Failing that, one could only hope that those preferring seclusion would have the luck to die of a stroke, or something equally swift, before the situation became too bad, for in such cases – or was this further evidence of the Doctor's unorthodoxy? – moving them into hospital against their will was even more cruel than leaving them in their squalor and dementia. They provided one of the more painful illustrations of the truth that, just as there are cases in which a patient must learn to live with his disability, there are others where a doctor, and particularly a general practitioner, must live with his limitations and his helplessness.

CHAPTER 14

RETIREMENT: 'I COULDN'T HAVE BEEN ANYTHING ELSE'

At one time – perhaps it still obtains – members of the editorial staff of a certain British newspaper, when they raised their heads from typewriter or telephone pad, were faced with a notice which read: 'IT IS LATER THAN YOU THINK.' Few ploys could be better calculated to make one perforate one's ulcers like a colander, but, opportune or otherwise, the warning tends to be well founded. It was rather like that with the Doctor's impending retirement. Traditionally, a senior GP's last few years in practice see him gradually tapering off his work, while, particularly in novels and television series, he imparts to his juniors the benefits of a lifetime's accumulated skill and wisdom and, in his increased leisure, looks back on the panorama of the years through a mellow haze of philosophy. If ever it really was like that, it is certainly not often so in today's conditions of practice. For the Doctor there seemed to be almost no transition between the stage when he was working his normal 12-plus hours a day five and a bit days a week and the stage when he was sending out rather more than 3,000 notices to patients which ran: 'In case I am not able to tell you personally, this is to let you know that I shall be retiring in September. Dr X, who has already joined the practice, will be taking over my work, with my other partners, whom you know. I am sorry to leave you all, but I know I leave you in good hands.'

In an area where, beneath one section of the population which was so mobile that a seventh part of the practice changed every year there lay another rooted almost as solidly as in a village, the news had sometimes preceded the notices, so that the valedictions spread over several weeks. Many patients – this was a phenomenon which the Doctor never remembered observing in pre-NHS days – brought or sent parting gifts, which might be a cherished pot plant or a dozen of chateau-bottled claret. There were children who would miss

176

his funny drawings, and neurotics who felt they were losing their prop and found it hard to credit how soon they would adjust to another, and lonely old ladies, not far from tears, who said it would never be quite the same with anybody else.

The last, of course, was factually true. One of the attractions of general practice for the Doctor, as for a number of his contemporaries whose abilities and qualifications would have enabled them to go what is usually considered 'further', was the scope it gave you to work in your own way, according to your own interests and personality, subject, of course, to maintaining acceptable standards. Sometimes the Doctor thought that the BMA would be better employed in keeping a closer eye on standards, as the medieval guilds watched over those of their members, than in indulging such a passionate preoccupation with medical etiquette and ethics, particularly when it showed a tendency to confuse the two. In the Doctor's view, medical etiquette, even if indifferent practitioners sometimes invoked it to prevent their patients leaving them for somebody else, was no more than good manners, plus some expertise in social deportment in the circumstances in which one happened to be. By the BMA's definition it seemed to be more concerned with etiquette between doctor and doctor, as when it was solemnly laid down which of the two should enter and leave the room first when one doctor called in another as a consultant, than with etiquette between doctor and patient. And medical ethics were just those of the Christian way of life: if he did not subscribe to those a doctor could not expect to receive, still less to deserve, the trust of his patients. In the twentieth century he could not see much need to drag in Hippocrates, whose Oath, anyway, had clearly been partly inspired by job demarcation – his followers swore that they would not 'cut persons labouring under the stone, but will leave this to be done by men who are practitioners of this work'.

Even if he had had time for it, the Doctor had little more taste for brooding over what might have been than he had for introspection, at which he was bad, not from any lack of self-perception but because he usually seemed to have something more interesting than himself to think about. Very occasionally he wondered how things would have turned out if he had followed his first inclination and set up in practice in a country

177

town. By now, he supposed, he would have become a rose-growing, fly-fishing worthy, even, time permitting, a JP into the bargain. There would have been compensations as well as the disadvantage that, in a small town, the isolation of a doctor could be more acute than in the anonymity of a city. When, at almost every gathering you attended, the conversation seemed to turn to medicine and, inevitably, one or more individuals left general principles for particular symptoms, social life lost a good deal of its attraction. It was not much consolation to know that it was probably worse for psychiatrists, or that the vicar was expected to show forth the virtues of respectability, dependability, discretion *et al.* even more conspicuously than you were yourself.

Sometimes, by contrast, the Doctor had speculated on how he would have faced the challenge of an industrial practice in the North or Midlands, where, if you could believe what you heard and read, the patients were man-eating. He had never had to practise against hostility, he doubted whether he would have been able to, but might it be that those patients were hostile because they did not think much of their doctor, or had had a series of doctors of whom, possibly with reason, they had not thought much? Perhaps, too, the attitudes of hostility between employer and worker which characterised bad industrial relations had spilled over into the doctor-patient situation. He would never be able to test that theory now.

There was one other idea with which he had played at times. What would it have been like to work in a mental hospital? Could he have maintained the detachment which was essential if you were to carry such a load while retaining the humanity you needed if you were to help your patients? Apart from that, he could never have contemplated going into any branch other than general practice, which seemed to him incomparably the most satisfying way of practising medicine. The conviction survived even his discovery, during the trough of the 1950s, of his father's fifty years' old account book, which showed that, allowing for changes in money values, the Doctor was doing twice as much work as his father for half the income. It would have been nice if the proportions could have been reversed, but even so he did not regret his choice. Almost any other kind of doctoring would have been rather boring because you so seldom got to know your patients as did a GP.

Could you be taught to become one, or, subtle distinction, could you only be put in the way of learning? It was a question to which the Doctor, intermittently, gave a good deal of thought, as teaching hospitals gave an increasing amount of attention to general practice and as his work in the Student Health Service at St Thomas's brought him into closer contact with some of those who would be the GPs of tomorrow. His first reaction on meeting today's students was that they were exactly like those of his own day, except that 15 per cent of them had changed sex – like other teaching hospitals, St Thomas's now admitted a quota of women. Closer contact revealed differences that went deeper than clothes and hair styles, both of which, he noticed, were gradually modified during the years of clinical medicine, to reach approximate conventionality by the time of qualification. On the whole views were to the Left of what had been the norm in the 1930s, and the students were more articulate and questioning, not only of accepted standards but of the hospital system and curriculum.

Back in the nineteenth century you had learned to be a GP by being bound apprentice to an established practitioner, before going on to a hospital medical school and taking examinations. The Doctor's father had started on his own by putting up his plate after he had held the usual house jobs. The Doctor himself looked back on his few weeks as a temporary assistant to Dr Vere, in the West Country, as one of the most valuable experiences of his training. Ultimately, the only way to learn general practice was to work as a GP.

Perhaps the answer to the question he had asked himself was that unless a young man or woman started with an interest in people nothing would turn him or her into a good GP, but that, given a right disposition, a well-devised training scheme could be extremely helpful. The Doctor thought that, ideally, every medical student, but particularly one who intended to be a GP, should spend three months on a hospital ward as a nurse, though no doubt it would be thought impractical because it would extend unduly an already lengthy training. He should certainly have a course in terminal care, which should mean a full-time junior appointment in a geriatric ward or hospital; it was not a subject which could be assimilated in a one-day visit of observation. He should learn First

Aid early in his training – without it medical students, even at the clinical stage, were apt to be pretty dim when faced with even a minor emergency – and he should learn it not from a doctor, but from a First Aider, who was likely to be a far better teacher.

It was common, now, for students, as part of their course in community medicine, to be attached to selected practices for short periods, and then, certainly, they had a chance to learn what general practice was about, though, the Doctor felt, least of all in the consulting-room, where, in principle, what went on was not all that different from a consultation with an amiable hospital doctor. The student should, of course, accompany the GP on his home visits, but he should go out also with the district nurse and the health visitor. He should spend some time in the practice office, learning about administration; he need not type but he should see what was typed and he should file records; he should deal with the home help organiser and the district nursing HQ, and he should answer the telephone and so learn something of the pressures on the practice and learn, also, to distinguish the fears and anxieties of patients which usually came out so clearly in their telephone approach.

Since he acknowledged the usefulness of such contacts and would probably have agreed that practitioners should accept responsibility for training the young entry, it may seem curious that the Doctor's firm never allowed student observers in the consulting-rooms. The reason conveys a good deal about their concept of what general practice should be. Within a two-mile radius of the surgery there were four teaching hospitals, so that patients who were referred to specialists inevitably had their consultation in the presence of students. The Doctor felt that there must be one consulting-room which was sacrosanct, where a patient could be sure of privacy and where, be it only for ten minutes, he and his practitioner were, effectively, the only people in the world. It was the factor which made general practice unique, and likely to become more rather than less necessary in a era of increasingly fragmented scientific medicine. One could envisage a computer which would make a diagnosis, prescribe a drug and give an injection, a kind of automatic consultant, you might say, only harder wearing. No computer could take over the human relationship between a doctor and his patient.

That was what the whole thing was about, really. It could not be taught, but you could be put in the way of learning it, and you never stopped learning about it however long you went on. Learning not to play God (here the Doctor was luckier than some of his colleagues in that it was never a role that he had cared for), how to prevent your patients from becoming dependent on you, how to spot the signs that you might be becoming dependent on them. Learning not to run out on them when they were unreasonable: in anything less than a matter of life and death the Doctor accepted that a patient had a right to refuse to follow his advice while still remaining his patient. Learning, also, never to take refuge behind a synthetic manner during a consultation.

'He always makes a personal appearance', said a patient of many years' standing.

Over nearly forty years the Doctor supposed that it must do something to you, but he would have been hard put to it to say what. He was certainly less of a Philistine than the young man who had gone up from Shrewsbury to King's: his wife had had a lot to do with that. Perhaps he was less of a blimp, too. Actually, he rather disliked politicians as a class and had never been able to identify himself with any political party. Perhaps he had loosened up a bit. Certainly, at sixty-five, if he had had a late call just as he was setting off for a week-end in the country, it would not have occurred to him to change back into a town suit as he had once done at the age of thirty. Still, he had probably been guided aright on that occasion. The patient was a horribly superior little boy who would eat no fish other than Dover sole, so he would probably have taken exception to a medical attendant in flannels and a tweed jacket.

He had stopped wearing a hat, too, though not as a gesture to a new age. It had blown off into the river when he was crossing Chelsea Bridge one windy day, and he had never bothered to buy another. After a few days he had stopped seeing the reproachful ghost of Dr Clarke-Foster, his bowler set square on his brow.

181

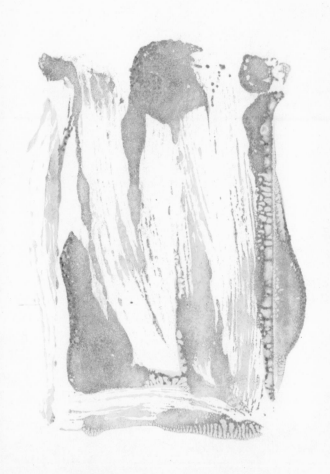